KNOW, GROW AND SHOW YOUR GRIT

Self-Discovery Made Simple

Hazlon (Haze) Schepmyer

Copyright © 2021 Gritty Guru Company

All rights reserved. No part of this book may be reproduced by any mechanical, photographic, or electronic process, or in the form of phonographic recording; nor may it be stored in a retrieval system, transmitted, or otherwise copied for public or private use without the prior written permission of the author. Send inquiries to https://growmygrit.com

Hazlon (Haze) Schepmyer, Gritty Guru Company

ISBN 978-1-7774299-0-4 (Paperback)

ISBN 978-1-7774299-1-1 (eBook)

Edited by Alethea Spiridon

Book Cover Design by Renata Chubb Design Communications

Book Production by Dawn James, Publish and Promote

Design and Layout by Davor Nikolic

Cover photographs by Ron Clifford Photography

Printed and bound in Canada

Note to the reader:
The events in this book are based on the writers' and other contributors' memories from their perspectives. Certain names have been changed to protect the identity of those mentioned. Any similarity to real persons, places, incidents or actions is coincidental. The information is provided for educational purposes only. In the event you use any of the information in this book for yourself, which is your constitutional right, the author and publisher assume no responsibility for your actions.

Dedications

For Sue Prior and Mike De Bonis who magnified the magic of mentoring at the University of Toronto Mississauga, formerly Erindale College.

For Nicole "Mama Bear" Patton and Kathy Swaile who facilitated the smoothest transition EVER as I moved from a full-time employee to an Independent Consultant for Team HoooooRaaaay in one weekend!

For Mom and Big Daddy who make amazing co-captains of Team Schepmyer!

TABLE OF CONTENTS

Acknowledgments 7

SECTION 1
Introduction 11

SECTION 2
Got GRIT? 15
   GRIT Growth Guide © 17
   GRIT Grid 20
   Phase 1: Know Your GRIT 23
   Phase 2: Grow Your GRIT 25
   Phase 3: Show Your GRIT 27

SECTION 3
Stories of Knowing Your GRIT 29

SECTION 4
Stories of Knowing, Growing and Showing Your GRIT 65
   GRIT Summary and Values from
   My Sweet Sixteen Contributors 141

SECTION 5
What Now? 145
   What's Next? 146
   Epilogue: Growing up with GRIT 148

APPENDIX A
How does Haze define her GRIT? 161

About the Author 165

Acknowledgments

In some ways, I feel like a curator and I want to welcome you to my first official GRIT exhibit! The contributors to this work of art, listed below as my "Sweet Sixteen", have shared their trials, tribulations, successes, struggles and setbacks related to completing and living from their GRIT compasses.

JAZ ▪ Janet ▪ Lesley ▪ Lyndsay
Drewery ▪ Moxie Joy ▪ Merida Jax
Neville Andrew ▪ Faye Schepmyer
Emmet Campbell ▪ Jennifer Neville-Lake
Mary Anne ▪ Elvera Guido ▪ Peter Charles
The Free Range Viking ▪ Catherine Noodle Wright

I'm grateful that each of you trusted me when I said that you have so much to offer others by sharing your experiences. Thanks for believing in my GRIT compass, for agreeing to inspire people you're never going to meet and for committing to something much bigger than any of us!

Special thanks to the May 2020 cohort of Power Yoga Canada's "Your Life Design" workshop which was facilitated by Pauline Caballero and hosted by the dynamic duo of Nick Vetro and Jess Moore. My 100-day goal in that course was to have a book in-the-works by August 27th, 2020, and it really happened! I am indebted to Marvellous Marni for connecting me with Remarkably Refreshing Renata who designed the covers of my book.

The number sixteen is also significant because it's been almost sixteen years since my first book, "Winning Reviews: A Guide for Evaluating Scholarly Writing" (Palgrave Macmillan, 2006). Although the format of this GRIT workbook is quite different from my first publication, both books showcase what's possible when a community of experienced individuals document their adventures with the intention of providing growth and learning opportunities for others.

My "do-it-yourself" GRIT compass is a tool for your journey toward self-discovery as well as self-exploration by way of knowing, growing and showing your GRIT (i.e., your default setting when navigating obstacles and challenges). Hopefully, you're ready for the journey and that's why you're reading this book! It's primarily a workbook that you'll pick up and start filling in immediately, then you'll put it down to reflect for a few hours or days, then you'll pick it up again to check-in with your thoughts and then you'll put it down again for new reflections.

SECTION 1
Introduction

My parents modelled grit throughout my childhood and being on Team Schepmyer has played a huge role in who I am today. Check out the epilogue for that story! A few months after starting my consulting company, I realized that I'm actually the fifth Schepmyer to start a business. My older brother, Anthony, has the most traditional company in the family and mine is the hardest to explain! There's definitely an entrepreneurial gene in my family tree and that gene was activated in June 2019, when I was one of almost 300 staff laid off from the largest Children's Treatment Centre in the province of Ontario, Canada.

After losing the best job ever, I decided to create the best job ever! In my opinion, the best job ever would be facilitating conversations that help people to know, grow and show their GRIT (i.e., one's default setting when navigating obstacles and challenges). Our individual definitions of GRIT will be specific to each of us and you will discover throughout this book that everyone's GRIT can have four different words or themes to describe its meaning.

I registered Gritty Guru Company in July 2019 and launched my website on October 31st (growmygrit.com). Two months after that, I decided that I'd get started on a book outlining my unique approach to self-discovery and self-exploration. My thinking was that a book would be the most effective way to share my GRIT compass with more people than I'll ever be able to meet through my consulting adventures.

My company name stems from my belief that a Gritty Guru is someone who promotes candid self-reflection and encourages people to consider the opportunities that often come with challenges once they tap into the mountain of resources already residing within them. Given that there's no clear end in sight for this planetary pause of 2020 (pandemic) and we're spending more time with ourselves, the need for constructive self-inquiry tools is at an all-time high!

Although the entrepreneur path I am travelling is new to me, it is defined by my commitment to my Plan A: accompanying others as they take the time to know, grow and show their GRIT. I've relied on my own GRIT more times than I can count since launching Gritty Guru Company and I want to acknowledge that everyone's version of tough is different. I understand that the challenges people face will vary in complexity as well as intensity. By letting others around me know my intentions, I've been embraced by a community of my own Gritty Gurus who have brought me insights and inspiration.

I look forward to hearing from other Gritty Gurus like you who buy this book and make the journey to know, grow and show your GRIT. Now, let's explore your GRIT!

SECTION 2
Got GRIT?

The first step in getting to know your GRIT is defining it with my GRIT Growth Guide ©. I use this tool with clients and its power is that it's always relevant and specific to you because you have to fill it in for yourself. Given that navigating obstacles is where growth happens, it's vital to understand the points of your GRIT compass and how to let it guide you over, under, around or right through the hurdles on your path. My sincere hope is that you can thrive on the opposite side of obstacles after you've taken the time to learn as much as possible about the strengths that you already possess and are bringing on your journey.

I shared my GRIT Growth Guide © with my Sweet Sixteen and asked each person to consider the same reflection questions I'm inviting you to consider after you've completed your GRIT compass. I received 16 unique compasses as well as stories based on each contributor's answers to some or all of the reflection questions which you'll find on pages 23-28. I wanted to capture a broad range of GRIT from a diverse group of people as well as a variety of strategies for knowing, growing and showing your GRIT. Hopefully, you may see yourselves in some of their stories and their experiences will enlighten, entertain and encourage you as you embark on your journey. Enjoy!

Take as much time as you need to complete the GRIT Growth Guide © then move on to the Know your GRIT reflection questions for deeper inquiry.

GRIT Growth Guide © (pages 17-19)

Sometimes it's helpful to begin a journey with a compass so let's get started on the path to growing your GRIT! When it's time to navigate or overcome a perceived obstacle/challenge, what defines your GRIT to approach the situation and try to get through it? What resources do you draw on that allow you to commit to an encounter?

Use this compass imagery to outline your unique G, R, I and T words!

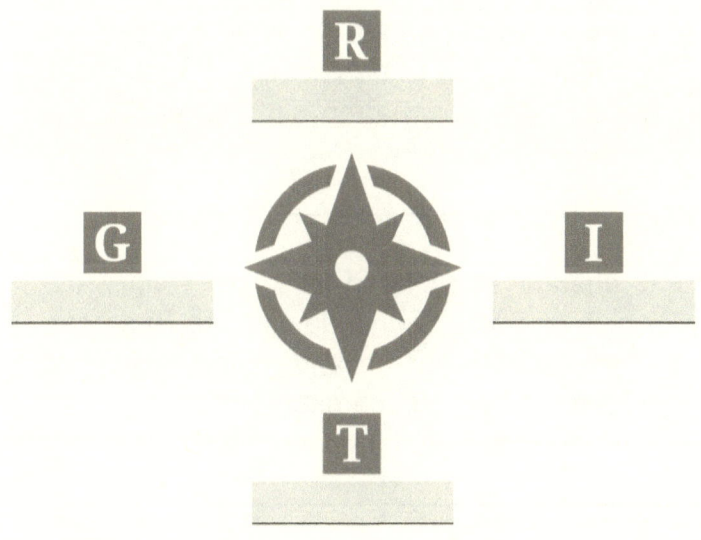

If you need ideas for G, R, I and T words by other Gritty Gurus then visit the URL
https://growmygrit.com/grit-grid

or check out pages 20-22!

> If change is required to grow your GRIT, which **three** types of change on page 19 would be easiest for you to consider and implement in your current situation/circumstances?

> If change is required to grow your GRIT, which **three** types of change on page 19 would be hardest for you to consider and implement in your current situation/circumstances?

> If change is required to grow your GRIT, which **one** type of change on page 19 seems impossible to consider and implement in your current situation/circumstances?

Change your behaviours	Change your intensity
Change your schedule	Change your mindset
Change your perspective	Change your routines
Change your relationships	Change your finances
Change your habits	Change your activities

Take a look at the following list of values and identify which five capture what's most important to you in life: https://www.guilford.com/add/miller2/values.pdf

❶ _____

❷ _____

❸ _____

❹ _____

❺ _____

GRIT Grid

G	R	I	T
Gas Light	Rings	Innateness	True North
Grid	Reservoir	Iron	Truce
Grid Iron	Rank	Incubation	Theories
Gamble	Respect	I	Totality
Guru	Receptiveness	Ideal	Tesseract
Goodness	Release	Ideology	Tapestry
Goods	Rabble Rouser	Introspection	Thanks
Garden	Raucous	Initiatives	Tank
Glimpse	Rules	Importance	Train
Ghosts	Risers	Inner Guide	Terminal
Girdle	Right Hand (Man/Woman)	Integration	Twists
Get 'er Done	Reinforcers	Ingredients	Turns
Gumption	Resourcefulness	If-Then	Tides
Ground	Readiness	Introduction	Tidal Waves
Greatness	Revival	Incandescence	Treasures
Giving	Riddle	Investors	Tingle
Genuineness	Reverence	Inventions	Tipping Point
Gas Pedal	Reference	Innovation	Tender
Giddy Up	Receptivity	Ingenuity	Torque

G	R	I	T
Growth Potential	Reverb	Invitation	Threshold
Guard	Rejuvenation	Image	Tolerance
Galaxy	Rights	Infinity	Tendencies
Guardian(s)	Ropes	Immensity	Team
Gleam	Risk (Taking)	Interactions	Trust
Gross	Riches	Interconnectedness	Trail
Grey/Gray	Ready	Information	Time
Goals	Resolution	Interests	Truth
Gang	Renewable Resources	Intelligence	Tenacity
Groove	Reflection	Insight(s)	Transformation
Glow	Relationships	Ideas	Thoughts
Go-To	Relations	Identity	Temperature
Generosity	Resistance	Intensity	Tackle
Ground Zero	Reason-ability	Insides	Temptation
Guidance	Rhythm	Integrity	Turbulence
Guide	Rechargers	Individuality	Tempted
Giggles	Reality	Intellect	Transition
Gratitude	Reserves	Imagination	Transfer
Grace	Reasons	Intention	Take (away)
Gifts	Resonance	Intuition	Test

G	R	I	T
Guts	Reach	Inspiration	Try
Glory	Rest	Input	Timing
Game	Resilience	Intimate	Tame
Grip	Response-ability	Influence	Thunder
Gather	Roots	Instinct	Tight Rope
Goofy	Resolve	Inhale	Travels

Phase 1: Know Your GRIT

The hardest part is now behind you; you've officially got GRIT!!! My next invitation is for you to reflect on these questions to complete the know your GRIT phase. Read each question and answer the ones that speak to you!

- Using full sentences or full paragraphs, how do you define your GRIT?
- How many times did you change your combination of words?
- How long did it take you to come up with your four words?
- If it took you a long time to come up with your words, were you struggling to come up with all four words or were you struggling to cut a long list down to four words?
- Did you check-in with anyone for help choosing words? If so, whom did you consult? Did you check-in with this person before or after you had selected some words?
- On a scale of 1 (not easy) to 10 (very easy), how easy did you think it would be to choose your G, R, I and T words? Why did you choose that number?

- On a scale of 1 (not easy) to 10 (very easy), how easy was it to choose your G, R, I and T words in practice? Why did you choose that number?
- What made you want to know, grow and show your GRIT?
- What was revealed about your understanding of and thoughts about yourself as you contemplated which words to use?
- What role do you think your values played in your selection? Do you see your values reflected in any of your words?

Phase 2: Grow Your GRIT

Now that you know your GRIT, it's time to develop plans and strategies to grow your GRIT. You may want to jump right into this phase or you may want to take some time to soak in your new understanding of what you reliably bring to a challenging situation. When you're ready to start growing your GRIT, I invite you to consider these questions.

- How will you decide which letter to work on first, second, third and fourth?
- Looking at the types of change listed on the GRIT Growth Guide ©, where will you decide to target your growth? If you don't remember, you can change your: behaviours, schedule, perspective, relationships, habits, intensity, mindset, routines, finances and/or activities.
- On a scale of 1 (not confident) to 10 (very confident), how confident are you that you can grow your GRIT? Why did you choose that number?
- Will you choose to focus your growth at home, work, school, rest or play?
- Will you have to give anyone a heads-up about your proposed plans for growing your GRIT?

- What will growing your GRIT look like for you? What will growing your GRIT mean to you?
- For each word in your GRIT compass, what is an example of what you plan to do differently in the name of growth?
- What will you consider for outcome measures or milestones to demonstrate your growth?
- Do you think that putting yourself in certain situations will allow you to grow more than one of your words at the same time?
- When will you feel a little outside of your comfort zone as you grow your GRIT?
- When/where will you experience growing pains as you grow your GRIT?
- How/when will you navigate your growth?

Go forth and refine your plans to grow your GRIT! Then, it will be time to show your GRIT. Fold the corner of this page, write the date somewhere on the page, put the book down in a place that you can see it and open it in a few days or a couple of weeks.

Phase 3: Show Your GRIT

Now it's time to choose your own adventure! You can start implementing the plans and strategies you identified to grow your GRIT (Phase 2) and then ask yourself these questions in the past tense to reflect on your journey. Alternatively, you can switch these questions to the present tense and use them as a final lens for making plans to show your GRIT.

- On a scale of 1 (not important) to 10 (very important), how important was it for you to show your GRIT after dedicating time to the know and the grow phases?
- In what other environments could you decide to show your GRIT (home, school, work, rest or play)?
- What was the hardest strategy to implement in an effort to show your GRIT?
- What was the easiest strategy to implement in an effort to show your GRIT?
- What reactions did you get from people as you started to show your GRIT?
- What reactions were you expecting?
- How did you explain the change in your approach to navigating obstacles?

- What did you learn about yourself as you began to implement strategies?
- What did you learn about significant people in your life as you began to implement strategies?
- What kind of time frame did you give yourself to make the changes?
- What do you miss about your old ways?
- What excites you about the options and possibilities that will be available to you one year from now?

SECTION 3
Stories of Knowing Your GRIT

Groundedness – Receptivity – Imagination – Tenacity

Practising physician and aspiring glassblower, 35
Loves tea, bicycling, yoga, and exploring new cities
Toronto, ON

Groundedness – staying cognizant of my existing skills, knowledge and support network to remain level-headed in new and challenging situations.

Receptivity to the prospect of change, to new information and to feedback/suggestions from others about how I might overcome obstacles.

Imagination - thinking about novel ways to approach a challenge when the strategies I've used in the past may be ineffective.

Tenacity in the face of challenges which may take a lot of time and effort to overcome and which may require multiple attempts using different strategies.

I changed one of the words once, replacing Innovation with Imagination. I don't think that there is a huge disparity between these words, but I do think that Imagination captures a greater sense of creativity and trying to step outside of one's usual thought process. It took me about 3 hours in total and I did not consult with anyone. I spent 1-2 hours coming up with a list of possible words and about 1 hour narrowing that list down to my final GRIT words.

I've always enjoyed word games, including coming up with acronyms to describe objects and situations, so I thought that generating a list of potential words would be relatively easy. I anticipated that the harder part would be narrowing my possibilities down to four words that encapsulated my strategy for overcoming obstacles without being redundant. On a scale of 1 (not easy) to 10 (very easy), my answer is 7 for perceived ease of selection.

Generating a list of possible words was similar in difficulty to what I expected, and it was easier than I anticipated to narrow them down once I really thought about which words applied to my personal approach to obstacles. On a scale of 1 (not easy) to 10 (very easy), I would go with 6 for actual ease of selection.

Completing the GRIT Growth Guide © made me realize that I usually start with a more internal approach when faced with new challenges – looking within my pre-existing skill set, knowledge, and resources – and then moving outward to seek new information, ideas, and inspiration from other sources.

I think that my personal values played a major role in my selections and are reflected in all of the words that I ultimately chose. The five specific values that I chose from the Personal Values Card Sort were curiosity, creativity, hope, autonomy, and leisure; in particular, I think that the first three are reflected in my GRIT words.

Giving – Respect – Integrity – Tenacity

Mother, Sister, Daughter, Partner
Teacher, Friend
Lover of Drake and old-school Hip Hop.
Lover of animals. I will build and operate an
animal shelter as my next adventure.
Lover of adventure to travel...I will see the world!
Mississauga, ON

I define my GRIT as my ability to GIVE fully with my whole heart and soul, giving and receiving RESPECT with grace and dignity, committing to being of INTEGRITY with myself and with others and showing TENACITY around people and circumstances that I believe in. I define my GRIT as my "why". Why I do what I do... even if it's difficult. Even after a great deal of introspection... Giving, Respect, Integrity and Tenacity... THESE ARE MY WORDS!

I love to Give and I feel that what I give to others is valuable and often healing. Living Respectfully brings me peace. Honestly, I love that I am older and that I can look towards my faith, culture and background to help me navigate this world. Being of Integrity is everything. Even though I may "fall away" sometimes, it's wonderful to have this anchor and this intention to guide as well as drive me. And Tenacity... I feel that my ability not to give up is my "super power"! Yes... I need to do some work around giving up "what I must" but I love that I am able to "stick with" the people and things that are the most important to me.

I am a total giver. I get the most joy when I am in a position of giving and I love to give to others emotionally, physically and even materially. Respect is everything to me. I am a first-generation Canadian and I have been raised as a Roman Catholic. Very early in my life I was taught that respect was everything. Honouring and respecting people, their traditions, family, and culture. It is all I know. Integrity is my mantra. I NEVER, EVER lie. I cannot. And the biggest offence I can receive is to be lied to. This way of being has often resulted in conflict for me. It's a very high standard that I hold myself and others to. If I am outside of integrity it "eats me up" and when someone is not being integral with me... I "can't fake it". Tenacity is important too. I do not give up on the people or things that are important to me. No matter how difficult... I never give up.

On a scale of 1 (not easy) to 10 (very easy), 10 is my number for both perceived and actual ease of selecting my GRIT. I was actually amazed at how easy it was to choose my words. It was as if they literally jumped off the page and they were all I could see. I did not change my combination of words even once because the choice of words was easy. I did not check-in with anyone about my words and, even after the above awareness, I love my words. I don't want to change them.

What came to light about my understanding of myself as I chose these words was interesting. Although the words are powerful and these words put into play should conceivably result in a powerful way of being, I also realized how living as I do can often be a burden, actually cause me pain. As a giver, I often have a difficult time asking for what I need. I say "yes, yes, yes" then often feel exhausted and spent. Then I can lash out at those I love and complain that I am not appreciated or supported. I often encounter "push back" from my four children and people in my life around my concept of "respect". For me... respect is a given... you respect your elders, respect the church, respect family and traditions ... almost unconditionally.

Some people in my life, particularly my children, may push back with comments like... "Why should I respect 'Nana' if I barely know her?"... or "Why should I get married in a 'church' if I don't even go to church?" It's a constant "internal struggle" for me; a struggle between what has been instilled in me versus how the world seems to be changing. Integrity is also a hard one. It's so important to me but there are places in my life where I'm not always integral. Do I always do what I say? Not always. Do I always say what I do? Not always. Ugh! Tenacity, as I said above, means that I "never" give up. And the result is that I sometimes need to "GIVE UP" on a person, a thing or a behaviour that may not be "serving me" and I won't. Not good.

I think my values have everything to do with my selection! They are acceptance, belonging, caring, compassion and contribution. At my core, I am very traditional. I was raised by very strict European parents. I have a huge extended family and all of my time was spent at home with my family.

I love the word GRIT. For me it's your "why". Why you get up in the morning and do "IT" over and over again. Your GRIT defines you, inspires you and motivates you. It's how you are perceived in the world. It is EVERYTHING! I am so excited to learn more and do more!

Give In – Reality – Input – Transition

Accessible Media Services, 40
Loves record collecting and record listening!
Toronto, ON

I've had a lot of issues with anxiety and panic going back years and years. Over the last few months, I've probably had the highest level of sustained day-to-day anxiety that I can remember. Since March 2020, I've taken another crack at mindful meditation and it seems to have taken hold. My GRIT words sort of align with that practice; they're 'Give-in', 'Reality', 'Input', and 'Transition'.

'Give-in' doesn't mean 'give-up' so much as it means accept what's happening. There's a tendency to fight against the physical sensations during elevated anxiety, so I'm trying to accept them. 'Reality' is about trying to step outside of myself and watch the anxiety or panic attack as if I was an outside observer taking an objective look at it, rather than feeling like it's happening to me. 'Input' is for accepting the sensations I'm feeling, but more as clinical data rather than things that are directly affecting me. In mindful meditation, I believe it's called 'noting'. I was tempted to change 'Reality' to 'Realign', as in realign the negative thought process, but 'Transition' seems to work as well, and I felt like 'Reality' was a pretty good one to keep. I try to transition the thoughts away from negative conclusions. That isn't to say I try to transition thoughts toward positivity, just neutrality. I try to let thoughts go by without attaching significance to them. It's hard! I find myself repeating the same steps of the learning process over and over again, and that's okay.

I didn't realize that the values I chose seem to be directly linked to my GRIT words until the question was asked explicitly. My values are stability, simplicity, self-acceptance, inner peace, flexibility and curiosity.

It's hard to know what behaviours of mine contribute to anxiety and panic. I've survived enough panic attacks unharmed over the years to have a little more perspective than I used to. Even if I'm in the throes of a pretty severe attack, there's at least part of me that clings to something sturdy and says, 'I've been through this before, and each time I've survived.' That helps to adjust my perspective and my mindset.

On the other hand, seeing that little light at the end of the tunnel never seems to make the tunnel shorter or any less dark. The intensity of the attacks is still severe, and the habit of focusing on the negative thoughts is a behaviour that feels impossible to overcome sometimes. As a result, the looming feeling of more panic on the horizon has probably kept me from showing more ambition in my professional life, and has led to a lot of comfort behaviour -- both of which have undoubtedly kept me from improving my finances over the years.

In the end, I still struggle, but I'm in much better shape emotionally than I was, say, 20 years ago. I mean, the pandemic's certainly not helping, but that won't last forever.

I'm excited for your new adventure. You are the perfect person to write this book, and this book is the perfect one for you to write!

Gregariousness – Rules – Intensity in Interconnections – Tenacity

Professor and Institute Director, 48
Mom to Draven -
my very own sweet sixteen kidlet
Loves football, gardening, and collaborating with Haze!
www.thewrightecotheologian.com
Indian Trail, North Carolina

I would say my GRIT is a story of the intertwining highs and lows, celebration and suffering, rules and innovation, systems and minutia. It is inching forward when heaviness holds my feet and blows hit my body but not my spirit. The universe put a love of football (nope not soccer) in my blood and it has always helped me personify my GRIT. To play women's football I found that you must have some level of gregariousness, rules-orientation, intensity in interconnectedness, and tenacity. The harsh conditions and the nature of this competitive game played with no protective gear was one of my crucibles for GRIT. I believed that my sole purpose was to protect my teammates and work together to achieve a common goal (score against the other team). We had a common goal, differentiated jobs, and a spirit of celebration that I felt fostered a keen sense of the rules and I felt their fracturing (usually in some violent way against my person) very personally. My quarterback was my leader and my team my family -- without question I rose to the challenge of defending my family --and even today I would walk through fire for some of my teammates. Football is a team sport that first taught me the intensity of interconnectedness and nature of tenacity. When I see or hear injustice today, I can almost feel myself putting on my gear to go into battle, knowing the cost personally and professionally but being unable to live and love any other way.

I worked on these questions while hiking in the mountains of North Carolina for a week, so I'll count that whole trip as my preparation! For numerous reasons, I think that I am constantly looking internally and have identified some of the characteristics that define me (for good or for bad). Thus, I think that the imaginative process of connecting words with feelings or aptitudes or essential characteristics was a formality of a long-time process. And as I evolve and am offered new opportunities, so will my descriptors I believe.

The words germinated easily so I didn't struggle with choosing my words. Where I struggled more was identifying the values that are most important to me. My top ten, not five, are: acceptance, belonging, cooperation, diligence, ecology, friendship, genuineness, imagination, integrity and justice.

On a scale of 1 (not easy) to 10 (very easy), I went with 3 for perceived ease of selection because I thought it would be hard for me personally. I talk myself out of things that matter to me or describe or impact the perception of myself. For many years I was told that I was not bright and that has a tendency to stick with me. But when I thought about how my daughter would see my words or another person who has been told that they are nothing or worse, I could almost feel myself dig in and drop my shoulder for this good work.

Using the same scale, I would choose 5 to rate my actual experience with selecting my words. It became a path that, once started upon, grew easier and more enjoyable!

I would say "yes" and "no" to seeing my values reflected in my GRIT words. Some of these are things that bubble up inside when no one is watching or I have identified as something I cannot control -- nor want to. For example, gregarious. It is something I have tried to curtail in some instances but when I am truly myself and free to express, this is a word that is at the root of my experience. It bubbles up and over and is essentially the life-source of my GRIT. It is communal, essential, celebratory, and relational which sums up not only my perspective in life but something so ingrained in me as far back as I can remember. This way of being has brought me joy and trouble! But I would not change it for anything. This is why it is my G word -- the first cornerstone of my GRIT.

However, I feel that other parts of my way of being also balance this gregariousness. Rules (and the essence of fairness and equity) is also a defining characteristic of my GRIT. This was the result of my interactions in the world, especially with a patriarchally-organized upbringing that was schizophrenic. My father saw to it that my brothers were above reproach for all sorts of abusive and destructive behaviours because 'boys will be boys' and yet, when a shed had to be sided or any hard work to be done, he called upon 'feminism' and put me to work outside the norms of women's work. Thus, in my oblivious youth I learned how to embrace the joy and darkness of what my gender entailed. As I became more capable and knowledgeable, eventually I rejected that which denied my worth and almost my existence. It oriented me to the work in Christian ethics that I do, namely fighting for those without voice or privilege. The rule I live by is simple -- just love. Period. What this entails today encompasses a minute to cosmic horizon of care and attention which takes creativity, deep listening and entrepreneurship to make sure the silenced voices across the divide of humanity and species are heard -- and they are loved. In the children's book, "Old Turtle" by Douglas Wood, there was a gem of wisdom that I try to live by in all aspects of my life: I am loved but so are they.

This leads me to the third cornerstone of my GRIT: Intensity in Interconnections as my I^3. I see systems of relationships in my mind -- the links and gaps and fluidity of movement between aspects in a system whether it is the pedagogical threads within an upper-level Global Perspectives in Ethics course, the multi-faceted approach to addressing eco-social crises or potential systems of relationality between our campus and community. I cannot help myself. It is a hard thing for me to get through a book without exploring every neat connection or footnote offered by the author. For me it is excruciating not to follow these threads -- I want to embrace the whole picture and not exploring pieces of the story is so hard. I believe that there is something beautiful for me to discover at the end of the thread -- it is like Muir and the mountains; they are calling and I must go. This revelation that my GRIT relies on an intense level of interconnectivity was important and it is also what I ask of others. I believe with every fiber of my being -- and personal experiential data to confirm this -- that resilience and GRIT are discovered and cultivated when one looks across human- and species-boundaries and we see how interconnected we all are. This must inform how we love justly. But I also have to accept that people do not see what I see and I must lead them along this path rather than expect them always to be treading this path beside me.

This last element hints at what I believe is my T word: tenacity. I cannot -- no matter how much I sometimes wish the opposite due to push back, doubt, misunderstanding, and outright hate -- violate the "just love" rule nor the horizon that I see this manifesting. I do get wounded and often exhausted. But I cannot help what I see. I do not see shut doors, just opportunities to take different paths that will be an adventure and a way forward towards a common goal. This is my general orientation and essence but this does not mean that I don't often become weary and in need of a recharge.

But when I reconnect to the source of my well-being -- genuine, reciprocal relationships, my family and nature -- I am reminded of the infinite timescale that the universe operates upon, my breath returns and patience is restored (albeit temporarily). I see this as a cosmic perspective of the very visual piece of biblical wisdom -- shake the dust from your sandals if the place where you are is rejecting you and your vision of justice, love, or life. I am a very visual learner and this image helps me find some closure and move on to another place in time where perhaps I will be more accepted or my vision of the world will belong and thrive. I also rediscover the innate bubbling gregariousness within me when I connect with the ecosystems that I inhabit far from the concretized and technologically-mediated world of suburbia. This brings me back from the brink of despair and moves me into a creative, problem-solving and barrier-reducing space.

Conversations with students and community members that I have had the privilege of working with over the last six years in North Carolina made me want to know, grow and show my GRIT. Even prior to the pandemic people were trying to understand who they are and where their GRIT lies in the midst of social, spiritual, and ecological upheaval. I work with people to help them to know and grow their value systems in order to act more congruently with what they believe and make the world a better place. This exercise is an important part of the interior movement that helps people thrive in our 21st-century world and it is my hope that these exercises will motivate people to ensure that all will be able to thrive.

Goals – Reason – Integrity – Tenacity

Seasoned veteran at seeing the positive as well as the potential in people and situations. Loves trees, dogs, coffee-flavoured water, old souls and art exhibits in small-town Ontario.

I define my GRIT by: Goals, Reason, Integrity and Tenacity. It took me about 15 minutes to come up with my combination. I didn't change any of the words after they came to me and I didn't check-in with anyone.

On a scale of 1 (not easy) to 10 (very easy), I would choose 5 for perceived ease of selection; I really hadn't thought about it before I completed the compass so I figured that it would be mid-point. Using the same scale, I would choose 9 for actual ease of selection because it was considerably easier than I thought that it would be.

In terms of addressing how I approach challenges, I don't think that there were any surprises or any changes in my understanding. My words just made sense given my past behaviours and my continued approach to obstacles/challenges.

I think my values played a huge role in the selection of my words; they are autonomy, compassion, courage, intelligence and integrity. I like to believe that my values typically guide my behaviour. An argument could be made that each of my values is reflected in at least one of the words.

Gratitude – Responsibility – Insight – Thought

Busy mom of two active boys, 44
Program Manager
Favourite things: Coffee dates, Zumba and
playing in the park on hot summer days

To finalize my GRIT words, I decided to take a specific example of a time in the past that was particularly hard for me. I used it to 'test' my selection of words one by one to see how that resource specifically helped me. Then it became clearer: Gratitude, Responsibility, Insight and Thoughts resonated with me.

Gratitude - Often when I face a new obstacle or set back, my immediate reaction is to complain and say this is too hard. However, because I've done a lot of self-help work in the past, I've trained myself to say immediately, "Thank God, it could be worse". I then try to look for the positives. I use Gratitude to remind myself of all the blessings I do have and how they can help me get through this challenge.

Responsibility - When I take responsibility for something, I empower myself to have some control over the outcome of the experience. I've realized that when I avoid responsibility, I essentially let the experience happen to me. I end up feeling helpless and live reactively, as opposed to living in a proactive mode. I can reduce my anxiety by knowing that I have the opportunity to take actions to get me through a hard time.

Insight - When I'm faced with a new challenge and I feel like I don't have clarity, I look to draw on other people's experiences. I know I can find someone or some knowledge to help me look at the situation from different angles. I fully trust that wisdom comes from experience and if someone has gone through a similar situation, I know I can learn from them. Their insight might be extremely helpful or only a bit but, in any case, it's more than I had before.

Thoughts - I've recently come to an understanding and true belief that one's thoughts can be the strongest resource of all. I reference here the Brooke Castillo model (founder of The Life Coach School): Thoughts have power. Thoughts create our feelings. Feelings trigger our actions and actions create results. Because our brains are always working, and thoughts are always running through our minds, the outcome of experiences are determined by our thoughts. The most fortunate part of this truth is, as humans, we can have some control over our thoughts which means we can intentionally use them to our advantage. This concept aligns with my R for Responsibility. I feel confident and motivated to take on responsibility since I know my thoughts have power.

When I first saw the long list of G, R, I and T words, I was expecting it to be easy for me to determine the ones that I use most often when facing a challenge. On a scale of 1 (not easy) to 10 (very easy), I would choose 8 for perceived ease of selection. I was pleased that I didn't have to brainstorm my own list from which to choose. I figured the greater number of words, the easier it would be! I had circled all the ones that were obvious to me but when I had to decide on the final four, it surprisingly became much harder. On a scale of 1 (not easy) to 10 (very easy), I would choose 4 for actual ease of selection. The whole process took me approximately 15 minutes.

My values are genuineness, mindfulness, inner peace, independence and music. When I think about experiencing these things in life, I can see a correlation with my GRIT. I want to know and grow my GRIT so I can show it to my children and be an example of someone who co-creates his or her destiny.

Gumption – Resilience – Integrity – Tenacity

Unique combination of young-at-heart and an old soul!
Loves the theatre, loves to travel, loves to spend time with family and friends.
Leading with my heart always has been and always will be my way.

Gumption, Resilience, Integrity, Tenacity are my words and the combination means sticking to my gut, following my heart and never giving up. I changed my words three times and it took me 10 minutes to finalize my four words.

My struggle with finalizing my words was more along the lines of thinking of words that start with those letters and then selecting the right one for me. I didn't check-in with anyone; it didn't occur to me to ask anyone for input since I thought that this process was personal and that I should select the words that I think are most appropriate for me.

On a scale of 1 (not easy) to 10 (very easy), I chose 5 for perceived ease of selection because there are so many words available and I thought it would be hard to narrow down to ones that would be most accurate. Once I started to think about it, certain words just surfaced easier than I thought they would so I choose 8 for actual ease of selection using the same scale. I think it's important for everyone to know, show and grow their GRIT. It's just hard to find the time to focus on yourself and really consider what it all means to you.

Through the process of contemplating the words, I realized that I'm stronger than I give myself credit for and am able to do anything I sent my mind on.

I think my values played a major role in my selection of words; they are loved, caring, dependability, family and friendship. I would say that all of the words reflect my values because they are who I am and it's difficult to separate that out.

> **Guts – Generosity – Reverence – Reinforcers – Integrity – Tapestry**

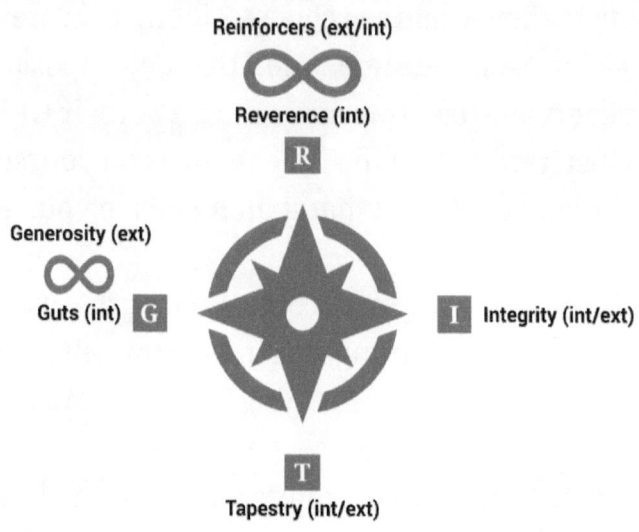

Broken-hearted;
frozen at 36, chronological age is 41
Nanay to 3 angels
Loves books, archery and music
Brampton, ON

I define my internal GRIT by Guts, Reverence, Reinforcers, Integrity and Tapestry. The external GRIT I need and value in others is Generosity, Reinforcers, Integrity and Tapestry. In my life, there are not just the internal factors like the desire to do things competing fiercely with intense fears and anxieties. There are also all the external factors like psychological triggers that are out of my control and that I have to deal with as well.

Guts - I think that every literal step I take is a demonstration of guts. My world is all torn up, with nothing being in the right space or place anymore. So, to borrow and paraphrase from Star Trek, my work is "to boldy go where no one has gone before", regardless of cost. This is internal for me because it involves a lot of mental prep work as each day brings with it so much fear, so many potential real-time nightmares and traps that I can barely bring myself to imagine.

Generosity – The gift of self from others – basically all the pieces of themselves that others have shared to help me carry on and carry my loves with me for the rest of my life. This external generosity includes: the messages people send me, the time people spend doing things with me and being with me as well as the spirit, love and compassion people share. I rely on it to complete my day-to-day activities and to navigate a situation for the first few times (or longer). Without others helping me through those first times, I can't do it. When I feel I am ready to try it on my own, then I try.

Reverence – I do my best to hold myself up to the standards that I did when my kids were still alive and watching me…because I believe they are still watching me. I try my best to honour and hold space for my loves who are gone and who are an essential, literal part of me. Science has told me that, as their mother, I hold a piece of each child in my body and all three live within me at the cellular level. Even though my loves are gone, what's important to me is that I always know, no matter what, I am acting and doing things that would make my children proud to witness and proud of me.

Reinforcers – This is both internal and external because there are so many reasons why I shouldn't do things anymore and a very limited number of external/internal factors that are motivating enough for me to try. My definition would be what I get for what I give and what I have to offer.

Integrity – Being true to my values and beliefs in every situation.

Tapestry – Every thought and action I do is a thread that supports a larger purpose and adds to a bigger picture.

I would say I probably changed my words about five times in total. As I was reading through each of the words in the GRIT grid, I first wrote down all the words that drew me to them along with what I thought they meant. Then, I looked up their actual definitions, wrote them out and renumbered my list according to those definitions. Next, I played with the words, putting different words in various groupings – and I always felt like something was missing but I had no idea what. I ended up choosing words that I was drawn to and I felt could capture a variety of emotions.

When I noticed that my two G words worked in harmony and so did my two R words, I started to wonder about a symbol for the interconnectedness among the pairs. I realized that the infinity symbol would be a perfect representation of how both pairs are integral pieces of my GRIT compass.

The infinity symbol between Guts and Generosity is short and chubby because those two words are fiercely intertwined in my mind. It is very hard for me to try to function with one and not the other in every aspect of my daily life. The infinity symbol between Reverence and Reinforcers is long and slim. Although they are connected, there is still such a gap between the two and I often struggle with finding reinforcing reasons for being here.

The placement of the R words was deliberate because reverence is closer to my core and matters more to me than reinforcers. This is also why the two R words are not beside each other – I believe that my actions are more purposefully reverent than done for any type of reward.

I didn't check-in with anyone about which words best suited me, but I did check-in with Haze after I had made my preliminary list of words. I asked what type of definitions she meant for the words (urban versus classic) and if multiple words could be used for each letter to make up my compass. I try to follow the rules as much as I can, whenever I can and since there are only four spaces on the compass, I wanted to check and see if I could use two words for two of the letters.

In total, it probably took me about 3 days to come up with a GRIT compass that completely satisfied me, and this includes the time it took to come up with the infinity symbols. I wrote the date on the top of my work and made a point of only working from that original list of words that I felt drawn to, working from my rough notes from the first day so I wouldn't get distracted or second-guess myself. I tend to doubt myself a lot these days so I wanted to see if I could create a process that, although was not flawless, allowed me to work consecutively and constructively on a project and left very little room for self-doubt.

I have been working a lot on self-discovery and trying to figure out my place in the world these past few years, so I figured this was just going to be an exercise in synonyms really. I thought it was just going to be that I look for a definition of the words that I think make me up and then translate those into the GRIT words. Before starting this work, I picked 5 for ease of selection using a scale of 1 (not easy) to 10 (very easy) because I didn't think it would be hard to choose my words that made up my GRIT.

As I was working through and trying to come up with my compass, I realized that I was intent on coming up with words that satisfied both an internal and external need for myself. I really struggled with the idea of trying to choose one word for each letter of my compass and, to be honest, this surprised me a lot. I thought I would be able to find appropriate synonyms that went with each letter. I am very good with words in a multitude of languages and I truly thought that it would be a lot easier to do than it was. But you know what? I was wrong and I'm glad I was wrong. It was actually a lot more difficult for me to choose the words that would define my GRIT because I realized that it is almost like I have two compasses that need to be balanced at all times. On a scale of 1 (not easy) to 10 (very easy), I chose a 3 for actual ease of selection because it was so hard in practice.

My values are belonging, friendship, practicality, purpose and stability. I see pieces of all my values in each of the words that I chose to define my GRIT. It's like each one of my values is a different coloured thread that weaves in and out through my compass and, just like yarn, it can be thick and it can be thin in places but it's still the same thread that ties everything together. I think of each of my values as helping to create and support the bigger picture, which is my life. So, to answer the question of whether or not my values played a role in the creation of my GRIT compass? Yes, I think they played a major role and will continue to do so.

To me, knowing, growing and showing my GRIT is probably one of the most effective tools in my personal arsenal of coping strategies. I especially like and appreciate that there is not just one GRIT compass that can be used for all things in my life, at least for me there isn't. I have the ability to create different GRIT compasses to help me navigate each situation as it comes forward. And so, I have created a few of them and there is a great comfort in knowing that I have these compasses, these little "Hazes-in-my-pockets" to help me as I move through the long empty days of my life.

SECTION 4
Stories of Knowing, Growing and Showing Your GRIT

Go To – Reassess – Instinct – Tenacity

Scottish Viking, 47
Currently wandering around North Carolina.
Dad to the amazing Kraken, and husband to Dr.
Viking. Loves travel and food and can be
found at www.thefreerangeviking.com

KNOW – Go-To: I tend to be the person relied on when obstacles happen, so I am accustomed to and prize being the Go-To person. Reassess: I have learned that, when running into obstacles, it is always good to step back and take a second look at the problem and at the tactics being used to solve it. It's easy to try and overuse methods because they have worked in the past. Instinct: I have learned to trust my gut when it comes to deciding on a new approach and in evaluating how my team may be able to handle a given problem. Tenacity: Call it Scottishness or Viking behaviour, but all obstacles can be overcome; you sometimes just have to dig in and do the tough work and accept that there might be some pain.

In my head over the span of a week, I probably changed my words dozens of times, but only once after putting them down on paper. I did it as a solo endeavour and I was able to come up with my combination fairly quickly, but only after a week of letting it simmer in the back of my brain.

On a scale of 1 (not easy) to 10 (very easy), I chose 5 for perceived ease of selection because I feel like I know myself fairly well and regularly assess myself in terms of leadership and strategic skills. I felt the exercise would take some work but not be overly difficult. Using the same scale, I chose 5 for actual ease because it took about the amount of time and effort as expected. I let it percolate in the back of my brain for a week or so and then took a short amount of time to actually get it down on paper.

I have really come to trust that I have good instincts when it comes to solving problems and finding ways to get things done. I'm stubborn, but harness that as a positive as I have found myself getting better at being able to take a step back and reassess situations and approaches and making changes as needed. My values played a huge role as they are what lead me in most of my day-to-day actions; they are adventure, complexity, curiosity, fitness and growth. I think my GRIT words reflect a lot of who I am and how I approach life, including the values that are most important to me. I'm not sure how I could have completed the exercise without it being a reflection of my values and thought processes.

GROW – When deciding where to start growing my GRIT, I looked at where I felt I was least developed in my opinion and made that the priority to focus on. For me, the main areas of focus are work, home and play. Resting is easy, but the other areas are all places I can improve.

Using a scale of 1 (not confident) to 10 (very confident), my confidence for growing my GRIT is an 8 because I have been able to grow a great deal over the past decade or so thanks to the amazing support of my wife and daughter and being provided opportunities to learn and lead both at work and in places like the softball diamond. Every opportunity to lead is a chance to grow, become more of what you want to be and increase the positive impact you can have on the world.

For me, the biggest areas to target were perspectives, mindset and intensity. Perspectives to push myself to see the bigger picture and be more empathetic. Mindset in that not everyone is a Viking and does not see the world like I do. That Viking mindset is an asset for me most of the time, but it does lead to trying to bend the world to my will at times, rather than slowing down and letting people develop their own ways. Intensity, much like mindset, can be a great asset, but knowing how to regulate it in different settings is very important and a work-in-progress for me. I am trying to grow past the days when I played softball and covered the entire outfield just because I was fast enough and because I wanted the ball more than anyone else. I find I work towards goals of this type better when I internalize them, rather than potentially creating outward pressure so I did not give anyone a heads-up about my plans to grow my GRIT.

For me, growing my GRIT looks like being better at walking that fine line of being confident in following my own instincts and digging into my inherent stubbornness without letting either of those become obstacles in themselves. Trying to ensure they remain positive assets by working on being able to step back and ensure that the approaches are right while ensuring that everyone is accounted for and given the chance to be heard since I have the privilege to lead teams at both work and at "play". Growth comes from not only improving the ability to overcome everyday obstacles with less stress and anxiety, but in doing so in a way that reduces stress and anxiety for my teams and simply brings more "fun" to the everyday.

In the name of growing my 'Go-To', I will work on providing more guidance and mentorship for those around me. For growing my 'Reassess', I will take detailed notes of my initial reactions and thoughts about problems/obstacles and provide myself with some time to rethink each step from a somewhat different perspective. When it comes to 'Instinct', I will continue to rely on my instincts, but ensure I am listening to those around me and internalizing different viewpoints to create better instincts moving forward. For growing my 'Tenacity', I will review actions afterwards to ensure that I am not straying too far into stubbornness as tenacity can definitely be an asset, but stubbornness can devolve into a problem in and of itself.

In terms of measuring my growth, it has come down to just giving myself honest routine check-ins to see if I am following the goals I have set for myself. Success will not only be reflected in what I accomplish, but more from what I can have my teams accomplish by being a better mentor. A lot of my growth comes from stepping back and either taking a second look before acting, or carefully reviewing afterwards for all four letters. The biggest discomfort for me is allowing people to take their own path to get to the right approach to a problem. I need to fight my instinct to simply provide solutions and instead guide people to finding their solutions, which also helps me become a better manager and mentor as I become more comfortable with things not being done "my way".

SHOW – On a scale of 1 (not important) to 10 (very important), I would rate showing GRIT a 10 because it is the perfect companion to concepts like servant leadership, and I think it is a great tool to create the types of organizations and relationships that can build the type of world we want to live in going forward. I decided to show my GRIT at home, work and play.

The easiest habit to develop/implement when showing my GRIT was assessing actions after-the-fact to learn how to approach things better. The hardest habit to develop when showing my GRIT was patience – allowing others to react and move forward against obstacles in their own way, rather than providing the "right way" to do things. Listening more, and developing more empathy. I don't expect anything overt in terms of reactions, but hopefully the reaction would be people gaining confidence in their abilities and changing their view of me as someone who solves problems to someone who helps people overcome their obstacles. What I learned about significant people in my life is that most people have huge capabilities and the capacity to overcome more than they know. The difference between solving someone's problems and working with them so they can solve them for themselves is an immense chasm.

The least sustainable strategy/habit when showing my GRIT is taking the time to look at obstacles and problems from different perspectives, but it is also one of the most important. Too often we are rushed into making decisions quickly or looking for the fastest solution so it will take work to maintain the ability to take some time and ensure I am tackling something in the right way. The most sustainable strategy/habit when showing my GRIT is empathy, as it brings so much to every situation, and the ability to truly understand what someone else is feeling is a great tool to have whether it be at work or home.

As I implemented strategies, I learned that I need to work on talking less and listening more. There is a fine balance between taking the lead and being a leader that helps people develop. Having the right answer is sometimes less important than providing the right process to allow people and teams to develop their own answers. I explain the change in my approach to overcoming obstacles with the following rationale: It is not about just pushing hard and forcing the solution; it's about taking a step back to assess strategies and involving more people to come up with better solutions.

This will be a long-term process for me. I have given myself through the end of this year to make the changes that will allow me to show my GRIT. In many ways, simply acting and getting things accomplished is so much easier, but the rewards for being more inclusive and a mentor are far greater and worth the extra time and effort.

What excites me about the possibilities that will be available in one year? The opportunities to have a greater impact at work and play by modeling great new methods and behaviours, and showing that you don't have to be the loudest at work to make yourself seem the smartest, in order to have the greatest impact on those around you.

Grounding – Resist – Inhale – Trust

I am creative and love making things! 40
I was quite young when I first needed to call upon my GRIT (even though that's not what I called it then)!
I enjoy being outside with nature, and sitting on a huge rock near any form of water is my most happy place!!
Ontario, Canada

KNOW and GROW - I wish I could organize my thoughts and responses in a systematic, question-answer format. In fact, when deciding to write about this section, I had initially decided not to. Who am I to say I've ever known or grown my GRIT? Oh, I guess I am!? I feel like a fake when I say that I can know or grow my GRIT. I mean, I have been through some stuff and, up to now, I have come out on the other side of 'that stuff'. Does that mean I have GRIT?. Technically this chapter *was* due three weeks ago… so I'd say it took me a really long time!!! However, I spent two-and-a-half weeks telling myself a plethora of excuses and tales that constantly derailed me from the actual task of sitting down, picking my words and writing about it!!

I hear others use words like "incredible perseverance", "tremendous courage" and "unshakable resolve" when they describe me but part of me just hears "blah blah blah". I can't argue with them necessarily and I can't honestly tell you what it was that got me here, but I can say now that I know more about GRIT, that the words make sense. I mean I wasn't doing any particular thing on purpose, and I don't know that I would consciously call on or activate my GRIT the next time "stuff" happens. Is that even how it works?

Before choosing the final words for my compass, I changed my combination about 37 times and avoided the task even further by making sentences for added effect! What was it again?....Grit Really Interests Them? Okay, okay, I think my words were Ground, Relay, Investigate, Time.....bawhahaha see, I am so bad, I can't even keep it the same for longer than 10 minutes!! Just kidding, I am happy with the following: Grounding, Resist, Inhale and Trust.

So, technically the act of actually choosing my GRIT words didn't really take me that long but please know the struggle was real!! Choosing four individual words sounded easy enough. Then, I would look at my completed compass and hate one word, so I would change it. Then that would spark a new word, so I would change that one, and then I would remember 1 of the 100 times I've used my GRIT in life and I would change all my words. This happened several times until I 'settled' on the final four! Ask for help you say? Someone out there knows me and could have helped, right? True, but I could barely get myself together enough to answer the questions, let alone ask anyone else for their input. It would have taken me another three weeks easily, if I had to sort through my thoughts and someone else's thoughts! I may check-in with someone later, but I needed this initial exploration to be a 'me' thing.

When it comes to understanding or defining almost anything about myself, I find it's never easy. On a scale of 1 (not easy) to 10 (very easy), I went with 2 for ease of selection. I think sometimes I make it through life by closing my eyes, putting my hands out straight and hoping I do not stumble or fall over in the first few minutes, or hit some poor unsuspecting person along the way! When it came to actually doing it, the task was harder than I thought and so I'd go with a 1 using the same scale.

Sometimes, when I think of something being easy, I think of it as requiring less work or less investment on my part. I could have done this quickly, played a word game, and come up with several words that might have sounded okay. Since I am on this honesty kick I will say that's exactly what I tried to do!! I tried to be all funny and say, who needs just one word for each letter? Let's make it a sentence and be all cool!! Get Real In Time, Gentle Reminders Include Touch, Generate Research and Investigate Thoughts and Growing Really Interesting Tomatoes, hahaha. Maybe picking my words would have been easy, but I find that whenever anything starts off easy, my brain finds a way to make it complicated. I often wonder if this is a 'me' thing, or do others do this too?

Like I said above, I like to avoid the topic at-hand and I use humour to avoid the reality of self-discovery. Not because I think I am funny, but because no one is looking at what they are supposed to be looking at if I can get everyone laughing. Also, when I finally told myself that this is what I am doing so it's time to "sit down and shut-up," I realized that there is a little part of me that is afraid to understand myself for fear of not being happy with what I find. I thought that if I labelled my GRIT, looked at it, and shared it, one of two things could happen. Either I would see that I have been faking it the whole time or maybe I would start to believe I had it?!!

My top values are commitment, imagination, honesty, purpose and growth. When I reflect on them, I think maybe they have been there a long, long time and perhaps, that's part of what got me this far in life. Subconsciously, I think that my GRIT and my values are intertwined. I didn't purposely look at my values and use them as a guide although maybe I should have! It's like a test from school, where the answer to question 5 is then part of the next question or even the answer to the next question!

One theme I can recall about 'stuff' in my life is that, in each situation, a fundamental part of me was being threatened. I come from a family where we were seen as a whole, not as individuals. We were 'that family'. We were 'the kids', 'the poor kids,' the 'dirty kids,' the 'stupid kids' and so on. I was often referred to as many other names by my parents and repeatedly told that my feelings, thoughts, and budding curiosity were wrong, were not needed, and were "not the way this family thinks".

So, as I got older and started realizing that I was an individual with my own thoughts, feelings, and ultimately, my own destiny, I became so very protective over that destiny!!! I was just a teenager at the time, but every situation in life from that point forward became about strengthening, discovering, empowering, and understanding my 'me'. Twenty-four years later, that's how I see it now. Still, back then, it was, "How do I escape from this sticky beast holding me back from the world?" Because I had no practice in the 'me' game, I think I sucked at it! I found myself in situation after situation that had me believing that I was not 'me' after all. It was so discouraging to feel the constant discord in my heart, to feel that "this is not right" about a situation or relationship but not know how to express that or not know how to resolve the uncomfortable situation.

I discovered that I would ultimately do anything to preserve my new-found 'me' which sounds pretty gritty but it wasn't! At times in my life, this obsession with self-preservation led to mistrusting others, constant quibbling with myself, a complete lack of self-confidence, narrow-mindedness and an inability to see the simplicity in resolving some situations. So, when asked, "How did you make it from that life to here?" my answer is usually "I don't know!" I can tell you that it was not from lack of trying to quit, to escape and render this life all done multiple times!! But, ultimately, my instinct for self-preservation won out and here I am today!

SHOW - I am a very visual person, and if I could picture myself GRIT-ing my way through life, I am imagining a person similar to a lumberjack, all sweaty from a hard day's work and wearing plaid like a boss!!! A big person, with eyes wide open and focused on the task, fully committed to the process and proud of his or her accomplishments. However, as I mentioned before, if I were to actually visualize my experiences so far, it's been more of a close my eyes and likely fall into a hole that appeared out of nowhere and tumble down a series of slides and tunnels until I come landing with a thud, somehow miraculously alive!

I think GRIT is like a seed, a tiny little seed planted in me. Maybe we are all born with it and, out of different experiences, the seed grows and changes along the way. When you're little and you have this seed, you don't know what the heck it is, maybe it's that apple seed you swallowed that one time, maybe not! One thing I feel like I can say with certainty is that this seed has evolved and changed. I know in my heart that what got me through 'stuff #1' is not exactly the same as what got me through 'stuff #2'. I am so curious to see how it has changed and evolved over time. Did all of it change? Did just some parts change? How far away am I from the original GRIT seed that was planted so long ago? Maybe, just maybe, I have a vast GRIT plant inside me, flourishing with amazing GRIT-fruit.

If I'm grounded in the moment, resist the urge to constantly second-guess myself, remind myself to inhale and breathe rather than holding my breath waiting for it all to end and ultimately trust that I've got this, then this sounds like my GRIT and I guess I have been growing it all along! I still think part of growing my GRIT will be taking the time to go back and understand my previous GRIT in the moments that 'stuff' happened. I have it... others have told me I have it, I have shown it... others have seen it. Ultimately, in the end, I think it only matters if I can find it!

The expedition has started, challenge accepted, the Find My GRIT adventure begins!!!

Genuine – Resonate – Ignite – Truth

Works hard to give her dog a great life, 44
Loves to find the perfect GIF
Toronto, ON

KNOW – My combo is: Genuine, Resonate, Ignite, Truth. I changed my words many times and I had a hard time letting go of some words that were close-seconds a bunch of times! Landing on "the one" for two of the four words required talking it out to land on them—I was stuck with two words that were true to me but I wasn't totally feeling it. I wanted novel words that really spoke to me. I wasn't totally happy until I felt like I had a word that really resonated with me.

There were a lot of second-place words and I had a hard time moving on until all four felt totally right. I ended up checking in with Haze. It actually helped to verbalize what I was trying to capture and then somehow the words just jumped out and the right ones were right without needless contemplation. On a scale of 1 (not easy) to 10 (very easy), I chose 10 for perceived ease of completion because I love words. Using the same scale, I would rate the exercise a 7 because it was harder in practice than I thought. I decided to know, grow and show my GRIT because I like a challenge. My values played a big role; I wanted my words to be a true reflection and mean something to me. They are compassion, creativity, genuineness, dependability and humour.

GROW – I just feel like starting now is always the key and that's the approach I took when deciding the order for growth. Waiting for tomorrow introduces a tsunami of things that will always get in the way. So the order I take to growing my GRIT doesn't matter so much as just starting something I can actually finish right now. I didn't give anyone a heads-up and I think this comes from being worried about failing and people knowing about it… probably another area of growth!

In terms of areas to target growth, work always seems to come to mind first but lately I'm trying to focus on play. In terms of behaviours, I decided to target my growth at work because it seems to always come first and it's easy to get lit up about stuff there. However, I reached a point where I realized that putting work first came with a cost and I neglected a lot of other areas of my life that became stagnant.

Using a scale of 1 (not confident) to 10 (very confident), my confidence for growing my GRIT is a solid 8 if I'm thinking of what I've been able to do. In the face of challenges, in the beginning, I'd say I'm closer to a 5 or 6. It always seems worse or insurmountable until I get started. When it comes to growing my GRIT and defining growth, I think it always comes down to feeling lit up about something; if that is there, then the rest falls into place. Growth to me is about always moving or working toward – I saw a poster in a lovely print shop in downtown Buffalo last year, I'm not sure who originally coined the message on the poster but I think it captures this idea beautifully: "Forward is forward no matter what speed".

I feel like I've got the perfect combination of words because they all flow together so when one grows the others seems to come along for the ride. Genuine: this one comes naturally if Ignite and Resonate are already present. Resonate: my tendency is to try to go it alone but I've learned that it is so much more meaningful to connect with others to achieve things – so this is a constant area of improvement; working on building connections. Ignite: even when something feels boring or insurmountable, it's great to carve something off that I can get excited about working on. Truth: This is an area of constant recalibration because it's easy to get stuck in stories or excuses.

When it comes to outcome measures for growing my GRIT, this totally depends on what I'm working on! I feel uncomfortable and out of my comfort zone (i.e., feeling like a fraud) when I experience failures or at least things that felt like failures at the time. Trying to distance myself from these things has hindered growth but it's so hard making space for painful things and just letting them be. I'm still learning and practicing this all the time.

SHOW – I felt a little disingenuous when trying to answer questions about showing my GRIT because I was interpreting 'showing' as 'showboating' and that's not really my vibe. Using a scale of 1 (not important) to 10 (very important), I would choose 10 for the importance of showing your GRIT. Lately, I'm trying to focus more on play because the work stuff seems to come together regardless of how much fretting and energy I give to it.

The easiest habit to develop and implement when showing GRIT is also the hardest... Just start! I'm not sure yet which habits will be the most and least sustainable – but I'll tell you in 3 months! I'm at the beginning of my journey (an action plan) right now and I haven't told a soul yet. I know I'd get support if I told significant people in my life, but I think I just need to see that I can get the ball rolling first and then make it public. The hardest habit is not buying into stuck stories or excuses which always seem to lead to procrastination. So just being really tuned into noticing my own snap judgments and thoughts in flight and whether they are leading me to actions that are going to serve my values.

I re-learned that once I commit to something it's ok; it's starting that is sooo hard. I had to take my own advice and just start, right in that moment and not wait any longer or think about options or wait and map the whole thing out, I just had to start. I've told myself that my timeframe is 3 months to start showing my GRIT.

It's nice to give myself an easy out. And I should do that sometimes, but when it happens every day then I'm not moving in the direction I want to go. Explaining the change in my approach to overcoming obstacles is such a subtle shift in perspective because all the barriers are still there if you start or if you wait and do nothing. The conditions and timing will never be totally perfect with an invitation from the universe to tell you when to start and what to do. For the year ahead, with my GRIT compass in hand, I'm excited about not having to spend so much mental energy on excuses and ruminating over why things aren't the way I want them to be.

Advice to someone who is interested in exploring the GRIT compass... Yes, showing your GRIT doesn't have to be loud and public, it can be totally private and still very powerful... but when you do show up, you definitely want to show your GRIT and not your s**t (all the stories and excuses of why you can't or what's in the way).

Gather (info) – Respond – Intention – Trust

A fifty-something young woman who lives in Ontario.
She loves NATURE, animals, and being outside.
She is a Christian who is married and has 2 wonderful boys.
Faith and family are what guide her life.

KNOW - I define my GRIT as Gather (info), Respond, Intention and Trust. I changed my words zero times because they came to me quickly and the ones I chose first were perfect for me! It took me 2-3 minutes, if that, to come up with them and I didn't need to check-in with anyone.

Honestly, I thought it would take some time to consider various words that would represent my GRIT. On a scale of 1 (not easy) to 10 (very easy), I chose 6 for perceived ease of selection. I didn't think the words would come quickly or easily. I thought it would be somewhat challenging to determine the G, R, I and T words that would truly feel "just right" for me. In the end, it was SO easy that I'd go with 10 using the same scale. The words came to me right away! No long reflections, no hesitation, no time spent weighting between a couple of words to decide which one would be just right.

I realized that, when I confront challenges, I do already have a way in which I approach them. Before doing this work, I hadn't given any thought about how I manage challenges; I just deal with what life presents. In choosing my G, R, I and T words I realized that I do approach things in a particular way.

My values are family, God's will, gratitude, integrity and honesty. My values relate to and influence my GRIT in approaching challenges. Trust is directly related to God's will. I trust what is happening in my life is God's will, that God is growing and teaching me through the events that take place in my life. This is my belief, what I value and what I trust in.

Gather, Respond and Intention are related to my values of family, gratitude, and integrity. Next to my relationship with God, my family is my priority. When I gather information and respond to a challenge, I consider the impact that these decisions will have on myself and my family.

Integrity and honesty relate to my intention. To act with intention, I do so with integrity and with honesty. I do not compromise my morals and I am truthful.

GROW – When it was time to grow my GRIT, I looked at my words and thought about which area would have a significant impact when managing challenges AND which area I believed I could somewhat easily make changes to grow. I decided to focus my growth at work and at home.

In terms of confidence for growing my GRIT, I'd say 7 using a scale of 1 (not confident) to 10 (very confident). I was pretty sure I could grow my GRIT, but challenging situations are just that...challenging! For me, I often respond from a very emotional place. This emotional response has years and years behind it soooo although I thought I could grow in this area, I knew it would take commitment, perseverance, and being very present. I was hopeful I could do it. My GRIT is completely interconnected so, even if I was going to focus on Response, I very naturally worked on Gather, Intention, and Trust as well.

Growing my Response (i.e., how I first respond or react to a challenge) would have a significant positive impact and I thought it was something I could start to do. Next was Intention. To manage the situation with Intention. To be conscious and in control of how I manage the situation. Next came Gather. I tend to gather information naturally however, with some challenges, the information I gather or consider may be one-sided and biased. Trusting was fourth. I need to trust everything will work out as it's meant to.

Overall, growth was being more in control of my emotions during challenging situations. Once I committed to growing my GRIT, I responded to challenges with more intention instead of reacting solely on emotion. I thought about it first and then chose my response. I gathered and considered aspects of the situation from as many angles as I could in order to get a broader and less-biased perspective. I didn't feel my emotions were running me. Instead, I objectively acknowledged my emotions relating to what I was going to do or not do. With a focus on growing these areas of my GRIT, I didn't feel the underlying panic I sometimes felt in challenging situations in the past and it was easier to trust everything was going to work out.

I found that Gather, Respond and Intention were very interconnected so they all pretty much grew together. I found that it took some work to remember Trust in some situations, but it was much easier to trust when my G, R and I words were growing.

SHOW - Home and work is where I spend most of my time and where my challenges are so those were the places I decided to show my GRIT. My experience was that the hardest habits to develop in an effort to show my GRIT were to be more self-aware and present more of the time, especially when I was confronted with a challenging situation.

As I implemented my new habits to show my GRIT, I didn't expect reactions from people to be different at work. At home, I anticipated that some challenging situations would be less emotionally-charged.

I didn't give myself a timeframe to implement my new habits. My plan was to begin implementing my new approach to challenges and to learn as I went along. I knew I would fall back into old patterns from time to time, but I wanted to show my GRIT by reflecting, learning from situations and acting differently from that point forward. I don't miss anything from my old ways of being! Everything is better and continues to get better as I grow my GRIT.

My advice for someone interested in exploring the GRIT framework/compass is DO IT! This is a terrific framework that is easy to use and is completely you! You yourself determine your GRIT and once you do, you go from there. So great! We all face challenges and having GRIT that feels right to you makes it so much easier to manage them.

Goofy – Resilient – Intimate – Tempted

Composer, Cartographer and Thought Adventurer, 44
Found in the Mountains.
Friendly when approached. Likely to deliver hugs.
Lucky Dad. Lucky Husband.

KNOW - I define my GRIT as: Goofy, Resilient, Intimate and Tempted. It took me five minutes to come up with my combination of words and I haven't changed them yet. I did not check-in with anyone because I am excited for this to be an independent journey!

Goofy shows up when I'm working to achieve the confidence of letting myself return to my natural self/state – which absolutely has a lightning bolt of silliness running through it. There have been prolonged periods of my life where this natural state was swept under the rug in the name of material/career/perceived "advancement". What a cost such a sacrifice can extract!

Resilience is refining my ability to see the forward motion/upwards trajectory when all seems lost – often it requires remembering to zoom out on a *massive* scale to be able to appreciate and see "progression".

Intimate is the creation and cultivation of safe spaces, emotionally and mentally. Intimacy nurtures differences of opinions and allows for emotional vulnerability without fear of judgement. It encourages reflection and the confidence to change one's mind. Above all, intimacy embraces fearless communication with the intent of betterment for and of all.

Temptation is a constant companion on my journey of self-*discovery* - which I don't confuse with immediate self-*improvement*. There are many side trails which have led to self-destruction but, with a map and intention set to self-*discovery*, I've been able to right the ship and return to the core path of discovery and learning. I'm always tempted by the mysterious and less-defined side paths along the way; this is what made me want to know, grow and show my GRIT.

On a scale of 1 (not easy) to 10 (very easy), I chose 9 for perceived ease of selection because the task, in my mind, *is* easy. The letters you have to work with are provided already – so all you need to do is supply the time to sit and think. Prioritizing the *time* is actually the hard part of this first exercise. I enjoy this type of work, I associate this with *enjoyment*, thus making the task easy and something to look forward to. Again, the hard part was allowing myself the time to sit and enjoy the process.

In practice, upon first visit to these exercises, actually choosing the words which represented my GRIT was not challenging. However, that doesn't necessarily mean I got it *right*.... The few combinations I could use were not difficult to discover – and there are a few combinations which make sense every day. I suppose to find four words that defined me *permanently* would actually very much be a challenge (and likely counter-productive) – but that's not how I see the growth/life process – these words are very true to me now, and upon a little digging have been aligned with my thoughts and actions for a long time.

As I worked through this exercise, the following was revealed (or re-visited)... I love words. I take them seriously even if the context is fun and nonthreatening. I also found myself contemplating the "What if someone else reads these and a) disagrees b) is offended c) would choose other words to describe me...?" In a nutshell, the perception others have of me is always peeking around the corner of my thought process.

For better and worse, my values and my personality are absolutely represented in these GRIT words. I hit them all very quickly and all at once. My values are: art, creativity, adventure, curiosity, intimacy and gratitude.

When I decided to try and gain some semblance of control of my life through "coaching", I put my own expectations or desired trajectory to the side. It was clear to me that whatever techniques I was currently employing were not successful. If I was to invest in the process of "self-help" or "coaching", I was going to let the coaches do their job. The easy analogy is sports – very rarely do even the most gifted of athletes succeed without the guidance and/or tutelage of a trusted coach. A good coach doesn't propose that he/she is *better* than the star athlete; the coach is merely able to channel and direct the raw talent. I knew this had to be the way forward.

GROW - When considering the areas where I could focus my growth (e.g., *home, school, work, rest or play*), my initial focus was *work*. Work was overwhelming, independent and unstructured. I was my own boss in a one-person geomatics department, but I certainly had to answer to senior management and customers. I began here because I thought, at the time, that this was where my problems were rooted. Once I could "solve" my work overwhelm, I would then be able to parlay this new freedom and fresh air into the other facets of my life. As it turns out, this was not at all what happened once I decided to get my hands dirty with some work/life balance and quality-of-life improvement. In terms of perceived confidence, I chose 9 for growing my GRIT using a scale of 1 (not confident) to 10 (very confident). I was very confident from the outset that change was possible but also very unsure of the path/journey and the timeline.

After hours and days and weeks and months of coaching practice and therapy, it dawned on me that the area of focus that would have the greatest impact on my physical, mental and overall health would be presence. I needed to grow my ability to be present. Not just in the moment, but present in all of my future decision-making which would also require patience. Presence and patience / patience and presence. They fit together. That's the behaviour I decided to consider changing.

I did not *have* to give a heads-up to those around me regarding coaching/desired change. However, I thought it would be helpful to talk about the journey with those in my immediate circle. In my experience, there remains an incredible amount of apprehension/suspicion about self-betterment, coaching and therapy of sorts. It is certainly not a slam-dunk that open communication of such a journey is guaranteed.

Using the 'Show your GRIT' questions in past tense, I'd like to address them as such knowing that the process, trajectory and goals changed over time. Growing my GRIT *did at the beginning* look like control and how to get it. I really felt like

I was being pushed around by my surroundings and being manipulated – so I wanted <u>control</u>. I defined my growth *initially* by how much control I perceived myself gaining back. This ties into the next question particularly – where did I begin my journey – which was work. This provided temporary gains and progress, but ultimately was not the core path necessary to real change.

My plan to return to Goofy is actually demonstrated in *confidence*, moreso than the *goofy*. This is an important observation as the point isn't to show up to life every day in a jester hat "just because". It is having the confidence to be natural in all environments and situations, which allows my lighter side to appear as it sees fit to appear – without fear of me being labeled as inappropriate.

In light of my Resilience, I am confident that change is possible but very unsure of the path and timeline. I am certain of self-betterment, knowing that this will be an iterative process and it will not always *appear* successful. I have experienced this time and again – whether through recovery from substance abuse, weight gain and weight loss, relationship CPR or music composition. All of these situations ebb and flow between measurable, immediate progress and frequent setbacks, sometimes subtle and sometimes not-so-much.

Intimacy is a bit of a crazy maker. *My* intimacy encompasses the whole of intimacy. For me, intimacy is real truth and discovery in all of my relationships. This does not mean that all interactions must be fire and brimstone debates and challenges; it merely means that all <u>personal</u> relationships must be ready to expose themselves to honest introspection and challenge. My plan to appreciate intimacy in the name of growth is to be aware and less fearful - nay – proud - of my commitment to embrace intimacy within myself and with those who are willing to adventure down this path. Self-betterment and perhaps betterment in general is, at its core, a very intimate journey.

My plan to appreciate temptation in the name of growth is Patience. Practice patience. Practice patience. The key to not following every temptation is patience. Patience allows me to practice my four pillars of patience and presence: Breathe + Think + Decide + Commit. There is absolutely nothing wrong with temptation – the trick is knowing how to guide it and that is a constant work-in-progress.

A tangible outcome/milestone which took a very long time to discover as a valuable goal is growing my ability to "de-escalate myself". It's not metrically measurable, but it can be measured inside. The beginning of my journey was often filled with distinct, traditionally "measurable" goals and outcomes – some of which were very helpful – however it is the constant challenge to grow my personal "de-escalation" ability that serves so many different aspects of my personal growth. Personally, de-escalation is also so closely related to patience and presence.

Practicing visualization and actually *feeling* the right decision puts me a little outside of my comfort zone. For example, being coached through a situation that demanded I stand, visualize, and physically step into the options in front of me – and honouring the *feeling* that this generated. The result was to resign from a 6-figure corporate sales job two weeks later and spend two months camping and playing with my family. The heart was trusted, and the heart delivered.

Breathe. The simple act of breathing allows me to grow and show *resilience, intimacy and temptation (patience)* simultaneously. When a situation does not resolve itself the way I had envisioned or an uncomfortable situation presents itself, breathing allows me to refocus and grow my resolve (resilience), look inwards and ask the hard questions of myself to overcome the present adversity. Intimacy with self and pause to consider the consequences of giving in to temptation of first reaction are my best bet before weighing all options.

SHOW - For me, I'd like to equate "showing" my GRIT with *"implementing"* my GRIT. What is very important to me is embracing and implementing my GRIT. This is a deeply personal practice and will help keep me in alignment internally going forward. I would rate implementation a 10 out of 10 for importance; it is the action piece that ties together all the thinking.

Interestingly, I find most of my "GRIT" occurs outside of work. I am all of my GRIT when being creative, or being a dad, or finding solitude – but seldom do I apply my GRIT definitions to my work life. That's not to say it doesn't happen from time to time – however I can fully unleash my GRIT in the other areas of my life that are less constrained by what one might call "corporate professionalism." I should think about this one a little more...!

Patience is the hardest habit to develop in an effort to show my GRIT. Presently, I am going through the phases of clinical diagnoses for ADHD/Anxiety/Bi-Polar disorder and have certainly been involved in various "help" programs related to these, in addition to substance abuse and mood disorders. ALL of these labels, which I am hesitant to use en masse but do so for painting broad strokes, have many traits in common – with the most dominant being impulsivity / emotional regulation / patience. It is *amazing* to comb through life with a new lens on my glasses. How does this affect GRIT and change and coaching? I want*ed* everything to happen immediately! And I wanted people to change along with me in the early stages. As I learn, I understand that these are not reasonable expectations. Patience is the key – and the door is often locked for me.

To be clear – my GRIT is a perspective of how I see myself and what I value about myself –but NOT necessarily what I wanted to "work on" in terms of coaching and development. I can see now that these four items would be enjoyable to pursue in terms of coaching. Because I was going in blind on purpose, I did not have expectations of others around me.

In general, I was supported for making the choice to leave a 6-figure job that was toxic *for me*. The job wasn't toxic per se – but I was ill-equipped at the time to balance life and the job. Through coaching, I began to realize that the job was actually not in alignment with many of my values or skill sets. These insights made the decision to leave the job quite obvious if I was going to begin trusting the coaching I was participating in. It was, indeed, the right choice. I received support from those around me for leaving a job which I wasn't aligned with – however many expressed their nervousness for the idea – as there wasn't a job waiting in-the-wings for me.

When I explain the change in my approach to overcoming obstacles, I say "First – breathe. Then breathe again". Just like Toni Braxton – thank you '90s slow jams. Second, I suggest evaluating how much of the situation is in your *direct* control then weigh your options, decisions and actions accordingly.

As I began to implement strategies, I learned that I need help implementing strategies (really!). That's what coaching and Cognitive Behavioural Therapy (CBT) etc. is all about – *I can, in fact, do this* – however I need a bit of help. I also learned that I don't need people as much as I am always allowing myself to. This isn't to say that they are not loved and valued. It is to say that I am in much greater control of myself than I was giving myself credit for. I was beginning to re-learn that I don't *need* people to make me happy and fulfilled, just as much as I don't *need* to allow people to become a destructive force in my life.

One simple example is letting a superior at work overwhelm me by adding more workload, extending work availability expectations or any of so many forms of "overwhelm". The reality for me was to address this head-on in a meeting. Reset expectations, ask for a few changes in workplace environment etc. and realize that, if these requests were not being actioned, it was completely reasonable for me to shake hands and leave. The alternative, remaining in a work relationship that was too one-sided, was not an option. My "boss" was simply my superior at work but not the ultimate "boss" over my life – which he had inadvertently become. This was likely not his intent at all; it was my own inability to articulate my boundaries and expectations that led me to remain too long and endure an emotional burnout.

In terms of time frame for implementing new behaviours to show my GRIT, I was trying to make little changes every week. The perspective that assisted me whilst trying this was: instead of trying to change completely or significantly in a very short period of time, imagine changing as little as 1% per day (a number which seemed reasonable). At the end of a year that's 365% (if that number even exists?!)

This was helpful – in helping see that small changes over a longer time can still deliver enormous results. So, I began to focus less on massive, immediate change, and tried to accept a "one foot in front of the other" approach and allow change to happen as fast or gradually as seemed natural. My first months of coaching, by comparison were all about massive, fast change – which was exciting – but not particularly sustainable.

As I continue to implement behaviours that show my GRIT, I'm not sure what I'll miss about my old ways. They served a purpose, for better *and* worse, and I think I am at peace with watching them fade as I develop *new ways*. Because of my T (Tempted) and my R (Resilient), I am always looking forward to new situations and new ways to *think* about these new situations. The "temptation" piece means that I am always curious – the "resilience" piece means I have a degree of confidence to try something and will survive if it doesn't work – and I love the unknown that is waiting – whether the unknown is a thought or an action.

In terms of advice for someone who is thinking about this work, although I haven't participated specifically in the GRIT program, I would *suggest* that GRIT is a game of "risk/reward". I use the term *game* intentionally – much of my time spent in a coaching environment has been (by my own choice) a very serious matter – but this does not necessarily benefit the coachee in the way perhaps imagined. As best as possible, be gentle with yourself during this process – even when making the difficult decisions and actions.

I would suggest that this self-exploration can be fun. Think Indiana Jones searching for treasure – *in your mind*! My coaching now bounces between playful and light, to insightful and mysterious, to emotionally draining – and this is all part and parcel of getting to know oneself better. Dig deep. If there is a "fit" between coach and coachee, you will feel it. Don't be afraid to dip your toe into the water of "going deep". It can be an exciting journey for the both of you; risk/reward applies to coach and coachee.

Time – give yourself time to ease into the program – and give yourself time to "recover". Just like an athlete who very rarely (if ever) takes on back-to-back days of 90% intensity – allow yourself time to recover emotionally. Even on the "lighter" days, I now take the afternoon off on coaching or therapy days. It allows thoughts to percolate or arrange themselves as they see fit while I enjoy an activity of some sort. Allow time for your brain and emotions to cool down and recover. It is fun, exciting, but nevertheless challenging work!

Go – Resourceful – Integrity – Trust

An effervescent, happy-go-lucky foodie behaviourist who is a realist and tries to find the positive in every situation.
I am continuously grateful for my partner in life, family, friends and all the blessings life brings.

KNOW – I define my GRIT as: Go, Resourceful, Integrity and Trust.

Go: When I am faced with a perceived obstacle/challenge, I will start by thinking and examining the obstacle/challenge and then come up with a game plan.

Resourceful: In addition to reflecting on past experiences, I will identify all the resources (people, perspectives, materials etc.) I need to overcome the obstacle/challenge. This is how I build my team of expertise.

Integrity: Be honest and truthful throughout the process to keep the process genuine and trusting.

Trust: Believe that everything will work out, trust my intuition, trust the resources and trust that if it doesn't work out, I will learn from it and alter the course of action or will do it differently in the future.

On a scale of 1 (not easy) to 10 (very easy), I chose 9 for perceived ease of selection. I thought it would be a relatively easy process to come up with my GRIT words given the list that was provided and knowing that some words would resonate with me. Using the same scale, I would rate my actual experience as a 7 because it was a little more difficult to pare down my GRIT words to one per letter. My process was to list all the words per letter and pick the one that held more value to me when I imagined a perceived obstacle/challenge in my personal life and at work. I chose the word that applied to both situations. I find that my GRIT words could change depending on the situation.

In terms of changing my words, I readily identified and picked my G word. For the other ones, I changed my word at least 2 to 3 times. I completed the activity by myself and I didn't want to overthink or overanalyze the process, so I went with the word that applied to both my personal and work life. Within 5 minutes, I had all 4 words. Although it didn't take me too long, my struggle was to cut down my list to represent each letter.

Reflecting on the words I used, I think I'm resilient in the face of an obstacle or challenge. I stay true to myself, act accordingly and rely on my intuition and others to overcome the obstacle/challenge. My values played a huge role in my GRIT word choices as they all further define/characterize who I am. They are family, genuineness, gratitude, growth and integrity.

GROW – Truthfully, when it came to deciding which approach to take to grow my GRIT, I went with the letters in the order they were presented. In a true situation, I would start with 'resourceful' as I would want to get the information I need to deal with the situation and access the resources I need to manage the situation effectively. I feel like 'go' is the next part of the process for me with 'integrity' and 'trust' occurring throughout. I define growth as learning something new, gaining a new perspective, using a mastered skill and applying it to a new situation. Growing my GRIT requires me to build new experiences, learn from and reflect on those experiences. Sometimes it isn't right away, but when I'm ready to do so and make mistakes as well as own up to those mistakes.

To say I only focus on one area of my life to grow my GRIT would be untrue. I feel that I'm constantly having to apply my GRIT in all areas (home, work, rest and play). My values remain with me and, as such, they constantly influence how I approach and manage different situations. In terms of my confidence for growing my GRIT, I would say 9 using a scale of 1 (not confident) to 10 (very confident) because learning is very important to me and if I stop learning then I stop growing. The reason I gave a 9 and not 10 is sometimes I just want to tune everything out and vegetate.

Here are examples of what I plan to do differently in the name of growth.

Go = to be more planful in the execution, contemplate more of the potential problems/barriers and come up with the solutions instead of readily putting out fires (more work-related). I would also add communication here as well given that 'go' still requires you to communicate.

Resourceful = continue to be resourceful and loop-in others, better communication system with others. There are times when I think about things in my head and forget to communicate it with others especially in personal relationships.

Integrity = continue to hold my values close to me and communicate them and articulate them for others.

Trust = I'm not sure how I would do this differently, but I find that I don't always trust my gut/intuition. Maybe I will let people know what I'm feeling/thinking and trust everything will be ok even if I feel as though there is never a good time.

In terms of milestones for growing my GRIT, I would look at my home life – communicating effectively with others and building a healthier lifestyle around food and exercise. I haven't quite shared the full healthier lifestyle with anyone. I will communicate it to someone as I develop a communication plan LOL!! For communicating with others in my personal life, the milestone could be reducing the frequency of frustrations I bottle up inside me and changing the number of non-passive-aggressive comments I make. For building a healthier lifestyle, it would be weight, frequency of engaging in physical exercise, the duration engaged in said exercises, and how I feel day-to-day. I'll have to figure out healthy eating

– but losing weight, inches, and feeling better may be good enough. In reflecting on all of the previous questions, communication echoes in all four of my letters. If I can continue to learn to be an effective communicator, especially in my home life, then I feel that the success will continue to blend into other aspects of my life.

I feel a little outside of my comfort zone in new situations (e.g., new job, new relationships, building new habits and attempting to change old ones). To navigate these situations, I go back to my GRIT to help comfort me outside of my comfort zone. From a behavioural perspective, I'm figuring out the antecedents needed to help me regulate.

SHOW – As I am using this opportunity to work on developing a healthier lifestyle, my responses will be in anticipation of using my GRIT. I am going to show my GRIT at home to develop a healthier lifestyle. I feel like the hardest habit to develop is keeping the Modus Operandi going and changing habits/routines/thoughts surrounding food. If I share my showing plans with others, I think people would be happy for me and supportive. In terms of importance, I think showing my GRIT is a 10 (very important). From a behavioural perspective, collecting data would be the easiest habit to develop/implement.

I would like to say to the universe it is possible "I am going to live a healthier lifestyle" and I am hopeful that all the habits and strategies I adopt to show my GRIT will be manageable and sustainable. Using a task analysis will help me maintain the skills. Through this work, I would like to learn how strong I am mind-wise to build new habits/thoughts. In addition, I would like to learn who is supportive of my goals and who are the sabotagers (aside from myself).

I would like to be living my healthier lifestyle in early 2021. I'd like to think of my indulgence in "unhealthy" food as treats as opposed to food items I should readily eat and choose over 'healthy food'. I'm still going to enjoy my lazy naps and zone-out periods in terms of things I'll miss because I'm doing less of them but still making time for them. In a year from now, I'm excited about how healthy and strong I will be.

If you're contemplating creating a GRIT compass, my advice for you is to "Just go for it". What do you have to lose?

Goal – Resilience – Intuition – Trust

Immigrated to Canada from Guyana,
South America, over fifty years ago, 71
Avid gardener and artisan
Mother to 4 and grandmother to 8
Loves Christmas, the Canadian National
Exhibition, snowmen and off-road cycling.

On a scale of 1 (not easy) to 10 (very easy), I thought it would be easy to know my GRIT so I chose 9. After having to cut down the list of words and changing my words many times, I would choose 7 because it took me so long to come up with my final four words. This led me to realize that I do not know myself as well as I thought!

My values did play a role in the selection of my GRIT as I see it. Diligence and being goal-oriented influence my goals. Having hope when it's time to achieve things relates to my resilience. Showing generosity, sensing the needs of others and helping them to the best of my ability stems from my intuition. Protecting and knowing what is best for my family depends on my trust.

I have not fundamentally decided to take steps to grow my GRIT because I feel that, at 71 years old, my traits are well-matured. However, I can work on my trust by learning to have more confidence in myself and not ask for a second opinion. My tennis coach often references the Nike quote, "Just Do It", when he's encouraging me to trust my intuition, knowledge and skills instead of over-thinking things.

When it comes to showing my GRIT, I would work on this in any setting although it would be a challenge not to question my decisions and seek confirmation/input.

Grace – Resilience – Initiate – Thought

Healthcare Executive, 38
Wife, daughter, sister, friend,
god momma to 6
Virginia girl who moved to Canada
for love, with GRIT
Oakville, ON

KNOW - I lead with Grace in times of challenge and times of joy; I have a foundation of strength and empathy through lived experiences which allows me to be Resilient; I Initiate actions and habits to add value for myself, for those I love, and for my community; and Thought will hold me accountable and ensure I do not stagnate and that I honour my values of integrity, kindness and connection.

Grace: *The quality or state of being considerate or thoughtful ... disposition to or an act or instance of kindness.* My definition of grace is embracing forgiveness, patience and clarity in actions and feelings; grace is love with kindness; grace is acting with goodness and compassion

Resilience: *An ability to recover from or adjust easily to misfortune or change.* A quote I have framed in my office is "She believed she could, so she did". Invictus was my father's favorite poem and I learned it during the 2020 COVID quarantine to honour him. Two lines from that poem resonate with how I think of resilience: "I thank whatever gods may be, for my unconquerable soul".

Initiate: *To cause or facilitate the beginning of.* My own definition includes taking personal responsibility to begin, to move forward, to take a risk without knowing the outcome.

Thought: *Reasoning power, the power to imagine.* I would also add the ability to be a contemplative person, to think and ponder out of caring, to evolve and grow through active thought about one's actions and beliefs.

When I started thinking about what was foundational to how I perceive GRIT and what has made up my GRIT, I started thinking about what in my life I truly remembered. My memories. Memories of what I know from being able to recall the real, raw feelings and environment versus what stories I have been told which formed perceived memories or stories.

I know exactly how I was laying on the couch in my childhood home on Monday morning March 18, 1996. I remember the sweatshirt I was wearing from the community teen club. I remember my mother walking through the front door, kneeling down beside the couch to tell me my 49-year-old father had a massive stroke the day before and he may not make it. I was in eighth grade at the same middle school where my father taught math. Every day after school for 3 weeks I would go and sit with him at the hospital by myself while my mother, also a public school teacher, was at home in the evenings tending to my 10-year-old brother and 7-year-old sister. I would do my homework, read to him, curl up next to him in his hospital bed to be close. Laying there the same way we had curled up the Sunday afternoon he had the stroke, which happened during a nap we were taking after I got home from a leadership camp.

I remember I didn't completely break down, or shut it off, or just carry on as a typical pre-teen. With poise, I would walk confidently by myself into the hospital and up to his room and then back down to get picked up when visiting hours ended. I did this daily until he was transferred to a rehab hospital. He had lived.

I don't remember my father, 5 years later, being in the hospital the night of my senior prom after his first suicide attempt. But my parents were sick a lot, so it is also not surprising that may not have stuck out to me. I saw him struggle through hard work and through motivation in rehabilitation those first few years. But real damage had been done – aphasia, loss of his right arm, difficulty walking, paranoia and anger.

I do however, remember his next big suicide attempt in January 2005, the night I got home from being in Southeast Asia and Australia on a trip to explore, play, and adventure after university. I had never gone this long without seeing my family. I ran into the house and upstairs to give my dad a big hug and kiss hello. My brother and I then left to grab a quick dinner to catch up since he had to go back to university that evening. My mother and sister went to return the rental car; for some reason our van was having problems. I remember getting a call just after we had placed our orders at Ruby Tuesday's that we needed to get to the hospital. He had done it again. He had waited to see me and thought we had left for the weekend to see my grandparents. He was confused by our plans and took all his pills thinking he'd have enough time for it to work this time. He had a plan but he was mistaken because my mother was only going to be gone for an hour. He had waited to see me though, one last time. I remember calmly asking for our food to go, not making a scene, with poise we paid and headed to the hospital. As the eldest of three, I needed to be strong for my siblings, who looked to me to observe my reaction and for guidance on how to behave. I had to be strong, I had to have grace in walking through the hospital emergency department doors to see him, knowing how frustrated he must have been to have been found. Oh, how heartbroken I was. He lived.

There were a few other times and it probably could have destroyed me. I desperately loved my father; I was his girl. When I reflect on these lived and survived moments, I think of grace and resilience.

My father passed on Sunday April 15, 2007, 11 years after his massive stroke. I was 24. It had been almost 10 months since he decided to stop getting out of bed. It was March of that year, just one month before his passing, I received a call from my mother while at a health care conference that he had stopped eating. Just weeks later he was refusing to drink. I sat with him a bit on a Saturday morning, knowing it was the end. My mother kept a cool washcloth on his forehead for comfort. I took it and squeezed a little bit of water out onto his chapped lips, his mouth so dry. I twisted the cloth to produce a little bit of futile moisture. He was barely still there. Holding his hand, I kissed his forehead and said that I loved him and goodbye.

My father's favorite poem was Invictus, by William Ernest Henley. It ends with "… I am the master of my fate; I am the captain of my soul." How perfectly fitting. My favorite two lines from that poem are "I thank whatever gods may be for my unconquerable soul."

I delivered the eulogy at my father's funeral, the eulogy for a man I loved, my father, who had killed himself … "our father was a humble, soft-spoken man, a man of relentless integrity, fortitude, **grace**, and character... we find comfort in knowing that our father is finally free. He was a brilliant man who had been trapped for so long. I think sometimes the human soul can only take so much, the fall of a man is tragic, and our father had a broken spirit ... we can only hope the peace he was looking for he has found" (*excerpts*).

To paraphrase Hannah Gadsby from her "Nanette" Netflix comedy special – "... I tell you this not for pity and I am not a victim. I tell you this because my story has value, *all of our stories have value.*" I tell pieces of this story, because I believe that knowing me, my GRIT, is to know these experiences formed the bricks to my foundation – a foundation I have built my life and life decisions on – consciously or sub-consciously. Not just my physical life, but the life in my head and heart which influence how I think about the world, how I approach situations, and how I treat others. Whether the Knowing is a friend, or me Knowing myself.

I rarely changed my words but I really wrestled with "I". It has been interesting to think through with the word choices ... selecting the one that is more encompassing, but not too vague so that it really honours who you are but not too narrow or limiting in the power of the exercise. While delving into these questions, I realized that I can frame "Initiate" as an active beginning to drive towards a desired outcome, behaviour, experience.

Because I think a lot through self-inquiry work (i.e., Thought), I didn't struggle with this exercise. It took 10-15 mins ... with the understanding that the "I-word" was still evolving ... perhaps up to this very exercise. I really tried to be honest versus writing what I thought the "right answer" should be.

I checked in with my husband and younger sister, who know me best and hold me accountable to being truthful, not just who I want to be or claim to be, but who I am – positively and constructively.

Over time through this exercise, I've checked in with my husband on my answers and how I frame those words to my experience and beliefs. In candor he has said my "I" could also be "impulse" and "T" "time". Both words with positive implications (although to be fair, they can also manifest in not-so-positive or constructive ways). Whether through my father's stroke or my health scare with blood clots, I learned at an early age that life can fundamentally change in a moment. You lay down for a nap and awake two hours later and your life and its path are forever altered. Or in love too, I chose one random 5-day solo vacation and initiated a conversation with the man I would later marry and move countries to be with. All this is to say, I can act in the moment because I have a keen sense of the preciousness of time. If I believe something will bring me joy, I am a very quick "yes". I always say for birthdays or holidays, I don't want gifts, I want time with the people I love. I want time with my family, my little niece and nephew whom I adore, my friends.

The beauty of this exercise, and truly thinking through your GRIT words, is it forces you to look at your core motivators and what makes you tick, what makes you "you". How you use those words to make a framework of actions and thoughts, what makes you uniquely human.

On a scale of 1 (not easy) to 10 (very easy), I thought it would be harder than it was when given the exercise so I picked 6 for perceived ease of selecting words. The "G" gave me a moment of pause because the word "grit" itself actually resonated, but then unpacking that forced me to really think about what it is uniquely about ME that believes I have grit in and of itself. Grace came to me in the context of compassion, forgiveness, and kindness. Having grace in the arc of my father's final decade. Taking that experience and having grace in caring for patients as a nursing aid while in university. Resilience embodies what I believe runs through me at my core. Having resilience to overcome my father's suicide attempts and death with forgiveness and strength, having resilience to hear at 21 that I had a genetic clotting disorder while hospitalized with bi-lateral pulmonary embolisms and a deep-vein thrombosis. The self-confidence and assurance led to really positive experiences in my life too through travel adventures, love, moving, taking professional risks, etc. The "I" work continues to give me pause between "influence" and "initiate" – Initiate speaks to me, especially in times of challenge or resistance, I move to action and control. In the context of a default setting of wanting to be in control, both words work (Influence and Initiate). In life this has been personified as the eldest child, in the professional success I have in health care leading business development and sales, in moving to a new country because of love and building a life with community and friendship. Thought came easily to me because I am a reflective person. I think hard and constantly about my actions, how I want my life to evolve, how I make others feel, how I can do and be better.

On a scale of 1 (not easy) to 10 (very easy), I would go with 8 for actual ease of choosing my words. What I have also been surprised to see play out over the last few months since I became aware of GRIT, is that my answers haven't really changed, except the "I". They haven't changed through the 2020 pandemic, through the internal exercise of questioning myself as the world wrestles acutely with race relations, as I reflect on the past but also what I want for the future.

I have a healthy degree of confidence but in contemplating the words, I also felt pride in my past experiences which laid the foundation for knowing my GRIT. I am always open to exercises that prompt and encourage self-discovery and self-evolution. The exercise can be a forcing mechanism to not only reflect on the past (good and bad), but also frame how those experiences live within you to cultivate strength and the undercurrent in reactions and actions today.

GROW - When it comes to the Growth, these are my intentions for each element of my GRIT.

Grace – be better at pausing when I'm frustrated - whether that is with a co-worker, my mother, my husband, a particular situation – and reframing my lens to patience and to actively work to see the other person's point of view. Not just a reflection on the surface of that exchange, but what is deeper behind it (i.e., the true intention, the foundation, and to have more empathy).

Resilience – take more risks and be better at embracing the unknown (i.e., less need to control so tightly).

Initiate – focus on outward giving back, volunteering, speaking out against injustice, actively engage in movements I believe in.

Thought – ironically, at this time in my life, I believe I should get out of my head more often and be comfortable and confident in who I am, the community I have built and not worry as much what others think or expect of me. There are bigger, more important things to focus on.

In terms of behaviours I can change, I can be less worried about what people think and I can be okay with falling figuratively and literally in my yoga practice. My inclination for 'Thought' is usually what leads me down the paths to be too concerned with how others viewed me. I also have the options to approach situations I cannot control with more grace and patience as well as sitting more in the present versus thinking so much about the past or the future.

If I had to choose one of the words to really dig deep, it would be Initiate – to be active and purposeful in taking a stand for what I believe versus being a passive observer. The actions though would be supported with the pillars of grace and thought, and the resiliency to be brave knowing I am strong but not perfect. When I think of growth and what it looks like – it is embodied in what

Alex, one of my favorite Peloton instructors, says: "Don't just talk about it, be about it". To be. The area of focus in my life would be in how I spend my free time (i.e., outside of work) and how I use that time productively.

I remember the night I met my husband in 2013; I was almost 31. Both of us were traveling solo at a wellness resort in St. Lucia. We walked the beach that night talking, and he asked me: "If your life was a movie, where in the movie would we be right now?" My response was "towards the end" … i.e., hardship, sadness, death, health struggles but she persevered – she was kind, grounded, loved and successful … that was the story arc in my head. I know now while that may have been a decent story, it was not only naïve but also short-sighted. How naïve to think at 31 that the hardships were in my past and how dismissive to my future that perhaps the greatest and most interesting, fulfilling times were not ahead of me.

At the very beginning of a yoga workshop called 30-Days to Level Up, I wrote in my journal: My father's death, his suicide, is not the most interesting thing to happen to me. Five days after starting the workshop, I wrote: "I can love him, miss him, forgive him but I don't have to live in the past with that experience as the defining event."

My declaration at the end of the 30-Day yoga workshop was: "My old way of being is to let the past be the prologue. My new way of being is to look forward with hope, joy, and patience" ... Growing and showing my GRIT is a deliberate and active change to the undercurrent and inner dialogue of my future approach, my thought patterns and assumptions.

SHOW - Showing is trying when it's hard, it is having clarity, and not caring so much who sees if I falter ... cultivate the self-respect that comes with trying versus perfection. I think of "showing" as truly getting outside of your comfort zone. To show is also to show myself, in the quiet corners, the actions when no one is watching, the intentions when you don't benefit yourself. As mentioned earlier, if "knowing" was an internal exercise, "showing" would be external.

For work, showing my GRIT would be a focus on how I continue to push myself professionally – not titles or a monetary chase – but building skills, taking on new projects to transform how things are done internally, influencing leadership and having a seat at the table.

For play, showing my GRIT looks like stepping outside of my comfort zone in yoga and cycling. Or finally signing up for that ceramics class I've always wanted to take, knowing I'd be a new student.

For service, giving back is a primary new "area of focus" for me. The other areas are current categories of how I spend my time and what I value, but volunteering and giving back would be something to add – to be active and deliberate in.

There is an element of getting out of my own way. In these last few months, I have focused on just stepping into saying "yes", even if it feels risky or vulnerable. And there is a spectrum, some baby and some big steps: I raised my hand to get involved in a local organization that helps stroke patients learn to swim and be comfortable in a pool (I swam competitively for 10 years); I was asked by our CEO to participate in a panel on allyship to the Black community for a company-wide webinar; I raised my hand to take on a new project to redesign and lead a national account strategy at work; I went cycling recently with two neighbours who are avid riders and I knew were stronger and faster than me – I initiated the invite, even though I was a little scared ... these are just a few tactical steps where I'm pushing myself.

This exercise and personal reflections are incredibly important to evolve constantly. I think it is also important to know what you can do and take on and what your limits are. For example, the last several years I have been wanting to find an organization to get involved in and give back to. And I'm now at a place where I have the space and time to really dedicate. But that doesn't mean I should beat myself up that I did not do it sooner. I remember in 2016/2017 when I was working crazy hours, planning a wedding, figuring out how to immigrate to a new country leaving my friends and family behind – that would not have been the right time and that is ok.

I see my values of integrity, kindness and connection reflected in all of my GRIT words. I don't believe you can truly have *Grace*, without integrity or kindness. *My Resilience* comes from living through experiences that could have caused me to be bitter or resentful, but I choose kindness and connection with people I love and respect. *Initiate* – this word only works for me if I know in my heart I'm acting with integrity to either influence myself into action or those around me. I also think there is an element of vulnerability that comes from "initiate". It is by definition a starting word, a word to begin. There are risks things may not always go as planned, elements that cannot be controlled. I believe being truly kind and building connection has to include elements of vulnerability. I have found as I have moved around, most recently to Canada, the true importance of initiating. Moving to the Toronto area, where I knew almost no one outside of my husband, I had to take initiative to build connections which I value so highly. It can feel risky when you are the new girl – asking a new acquaintance to coffee or to lunch, seeing if folks wanted to go on a walk – to create moments to build connection to lead to friendship. And finally Thought. I chose this word because I am deliberate in action and that comes from deliberate thought. *Thought* in how actions will make others feel, thought in how certain actions, or inaction, will result in achieving a goal or intention, thought around "why" I do or believe certain things. Thought and internal dialogue to constantly check myself – "am I acting with integrity, am I being truly kind or just nice, am I building honest and trustworthy connections?"

Knowing my GRIT has been an internal exercise, pivotal life moments that have created this foundation. My goal in growing my GRIT is for the work to evolve purposely with external-facing intention. Be patient with yourself while not being complacent would be my biggest piece of advice for someone who wants to create and live from your GRIT compass.

GRIT Summary and Values from My Sweet Sixteen Contributors

G	R	I	T	Values
Gather (information)	Respond	Intention	Trust	Family, God's Will, Gratitude, Integrity, Honesty
Gumption	Resilience	Integrity	Tenacity	Loved, Caring, Dependability, Family, Friendship
Gratitude	Responsibility	Insight	Thoughts	Genuineness, Mindfulness, Inner Peace, Independence, Music
Give-in	Reality	Input	Transition	Stability, Simplicity, Self-Acceptance, Inner Peace, Flexibility, Curiosity
Groundedness	Receptivity	Imagination	Tenacity	Curiosity, Creativity, Hope, Autonomy, Leisure

G	R	I	T	Values
Goals	Resilience	Intuition	Trust	Hope, Protect, Family, Diligence, Generosity
Generosity	Reinforcers	Integrity	Tapestry	Belonging, Friendship, Practicality, Purpose, Stability
Guts	Reverence	Integrity	Tapestry	
Grace	Resilience	Influence	Thought	Integrity, Kindness, Connection
Goofy	Resilient	Intimate	Tempted	Art, Creativity, Adventure, Curiosity, Intimacy, Gratitude
Gregarious	Rules	Intensity in Interconnections	Tenacity	Acceptance, Belonging, Cooperation, Diligence, Ecology, Friendship, Genuineness, Imagination, Integrity, Justice
Go	Resourceful	Integrity	Trust	Family, Genuineness, Gratitude, Growth, Integrity

G	R	I	T	Values
Go-To	Reassess	Instinct	Tenacity	Adventure, Complexity, Curiosity, Fitness, Growth
Genuine	Resonate	Ignite	Truth	Compassion, Creativity, Genuineness, Dependability, Humour
Goals	Reason	Integrity	Tenacity	Autonomy, Compassion, Courage, Intelligence, Integrity
Grounding	Resist	Inhale	Trust	Commitment, Imagination, Honesty, Purpose, Growth
Giving	Respect	Integrity	Tenacity	Acceptance, Belonging, Caring, Compassion, Contribution

SECTION 5
What Now?

Hello again!

Looking back, I offered you my GRIT Growth Guide © as an accessible self-discovery tool and explained how you can use your unique compass to know, grow and show your GRIT. Then, I shared the trials, tribulations, successes, struggles and setbacks that 16 diverse people had as they got to know, grow and show their GRIT. Next, you did the work and you made it into the community of GRITizens – people who know how to grow and show their GRIT.

Now that you've made the journey, which of the following is true for you?

- You have access to a trusted tool and you're going to use it for different contexts and phases in your life.
- You believed in your abilities to navigate an obstacle, but you weren't sure where to start. This GRIT workbook has given you the chance to consider past experiences that clearly support your ability to approach obstacles in the future.
- You've done a bit of self-discovery and self-exploration in the past and you appreciate this novel way to bundle your skills.
- Going forward, you're committed to approaching self-discovery and self-exploration with renewed passion and purpose. In addition, you've reconnected with the idea of opportunities on the other side of an obstacle.

What's Next?

Let's stay connected!

Follow me on Instagram and Facebook (@growmygrit)

- Engage me as a guest speaker for in-person and online events
- Book me to develop and deliver customized workshops for your group (in-person or online)
- Work with me in-person or online to dig deeper into your individual GRIT compass. Together we will:
  - explore the ways your G, R, I and T words connect, compete and/or cooperate
  - reflect on your struggles and successes in order to learn from them
  - make plans to navigate existing and upcoming obstacles while balancing effort and ease

For those of you who don't feel like you heard enough about me, check out the epilogue and Appendix A for stories on where I got my GRIT and how I define it!

You can also learn more at growmygrit.com.

Epilogue: Growing up with GRIT

I asked my Mom to write a chapter for this book, with insights from my Dad, because people always ask me where I got my GRIT.

I can say with complete confidence that my parents modeled grit for me, my three siblings, my cousins, my friends, their own siblings, their own friends and our neighbours.

For the epilogue, I took the liberty of pulling out the main themes from my Mom's chapter and organizing them into a GRIT compass for my childhood. The four themes are:
1. Get educated
2. Remember your rights
3. Invest in adventure
4. Team Schepmyer ROCKS!

Take it away Mom!

Get Educated

My husband and I are from Guyanese families in which the value of education was emphasized for children. We taught our own children at a very young age that we would not give rewards for good grades. We were very clear that the purpose of succeeding in school was to gain the knowledge and skills needed for a productive, successful and hopefully, happy life. Good grades were not contingent on rewards or bribes. Our oldest son, Anthony, grew up in Guyana and immigrated to Canada in his twenties; he instilled the same values in his three boys.

It was very important to us that we attend every parent-teacher interview, although we were once told by one of Hazlon's primary school teachers we did not need to attend because she could become whatever she wanted. I did inform him that we expected them to continue scheduling interviews for her because she would eventually experience her first rejection/failure in the real-world and we would be there for her. We also wanted her to understand that things don't always work out as planned because there are times when there is a bigger plan in place. *Author's note: Thank you, Mr. Luxton, for your faith in my abilities and for teaching us cancellation questions!!!*

Throughout school, Hazlon had been identified as intellectually gifted and was always in programs that offered accelerated learning opportunities for its students. It all started when she was three-and-a-half years old and her preschool teacher, Mrs. Schuller, recognized her intellectual gift. She suggested we investigate the possibility of her starting primary school at four years old. We pursued this with the public school board but were told that at four she would not be socially mature enough to be with five-year-olds. *Author's note: I often refer to myself as the tallest six-year-old you'll ever meet so I definitely feel less mature than most of my friends!*

In considering fun activities that exposed the children to different spaces, we had picnics on the grounds of the University of Toronto's St. George Campus when the girls were about seven and eight years old. I felt that knowing about higher learning, being surrounded by energetic youth and seeing history as well as architecture would be beneficial in making the children comfortable in such a space. I guess it did, because our three Canadian-born-and-raised children attended the University of Toronto. Hazlon was the Valedictorian of her class at the University of Toronto Mississauga (UTM) in 2000. Seven years later, she received one of UTM's inaugural Top Alumni awards recognizing the 40 most outstanding alumni when UTM celebrated its 40th anniversary.

Recognize your Rights

My husband and I wanted very much to prepare our children should they encounter some of the challenges we faced because we are Black. I can recall many memorable situations that provided our children with a sense of confidence to be comfortable in situations where they were made to feel like they didn't belong.

Sending them to school on public transit in the 1980s offered some opportunities for the girls to witness our support for them and gain tools to feel empowered to handle certain situations. Two examples come to mind; the first involved a bus driver smoking on the bus at a GO station, which at the time was allowed because it was a break-time. The girls, who usually sat close to the front of the bus, expressed some discomfort at the cigarette smoke and were told to go to the back of the bus. Of course, when I heard this phrase being used to young Black girls, I was angry. I called Mississauga Transit's head office to complain and that is when I learned smoking was permitted at designated stops. I appreciated the explanation but I made it clear that, based on the history of that phrase, you do not tell a Black person to "go to the back of the bus". I did receive an apology and was told there would be some sensitivity training.

A second example is when they were asked by a passenger to move from where they were seated because she always sat there. I did let them know they did not have to move because, like her, they paid to ride that bus and were free to choose where to sit unless the company designated specific seats to accommodate passengers with varying accessibility and mobility needs.

As our children continued to meet people who would try to stand in their way or set unrealistic expectations, our children were strong in the knowledge of our continued support. This was evident again when Hazlon, who has always been fiercely committed to her sports team, sustained a stress fracture in her posterior right tibial cortex during high school. She was still expected to participate in regional competitions but we let her coach know that she would not need a sports scholarship to succeed in this world. She would make it with her brains and our support even if it meant us having to work extra hours at extra jobs. At the end of the season, it made us happy when her team members voted her Most Valuable Player even though her contribution was cut short that year.

Our youngest son, Andrew, decided at age nine that he wanted to learn Mandarin through a program available to Mississauga residents. The first challenge was when the Program Administrator, a White male, wanted to know why we were registering Andrew in this program. I did explain our reason, but the Program Administrator commented that students in these programs usually belong to the specific cultural groups associated with the language. I did inform him that as long as Andrew wanted to be there, he will be there and we will support him. When I took Andrew to his kindergarten classroom, I was questioned again about why he was there. At this point, I was obviously not pleased with these questions. As calmly as possible, I repeated that my taxes were paying for this program and, as long as he wanted to be there, he would participate. When I went to meet him at the end of his first class, I received many questioning looks, was asked if my child's father was Chinese and asked again why he wanted to learn Mandarin. I recognized the need for ongoing support through the early years of this language program so I would crochet or read in the school's cafeteria in case Andrew needed me for any reason.

Andrew was the only non-Asian child in the entire program of almost 400 students up to grade 12; he was also the oldest in his kindergarten class. Because Andrew was so comfortable in taking his seat and learning a new language, I realized that exposing our children to so much variety and letting them know we will be there to support them was paying off.

Since Mandarin was not spoken in our home, Andrew did take private lessons from grade 2 until grade 12. As it turned out, Mandarin benefited Andrew in ways we did not foresee. In addition to being his only arts credit in high school, we feel his fluency with languages played a role in his admission to medical school. One member of his interview panel asked him a question in Mandarin and another asked him a question in French. We feel that Andrew's ability to communicate in three languages during his interview separated him from other candidates because it showed the breadth, depth and unique nature of his interests.

Invest in Adventure

We made the decision that, as parents raising two Black females in North America in the 1970s and 1980s, we would give them every opportunity to succeed and be well-rounded even through our years of under-employment.

At a young age, both Hazlon and Nevella played soft lacrosse. Hazlon always approached things with a "no fear" attitude and sports were no exception; she quickly moved over to full-contact box lacrosse with the boys. She typically played goalie and amazed the opposing team when she took off her helmet and they saw her bows in her hair. Hazlon continued playing box lacrosse with travel teams, and our family enjoyed the benefit of billeting visiting team members from other provinces. She also had the opportunity to travel through Europe (Italy, Germany, Switzerland and Austria) with her high school field hockey team.

Another avenue we took to help develop their well-roundedness was exposing them to activities where we were the only Blacks present, such as camping in Bruce Peninsula National Park. We started doing this in 1985 while I was pregnant with Andrew; we would take the MS Chi-Cheemaun ferry across to Manitoulin Island and then drive to Mikisew Provincial Park outside of North Bay. During those years, although we did not see other Black families engaged in this activity, we continued doing it because of the positive experiences. There are so many lessons we took time to teach our children either directly or indirectly while on these adventures: have a sense of purpose, walk with a purpose, care for others and share with others. In learning to care for others, our children were always taught to try to befriend, speak to and include peers who were left out for whatever reason.

A significant benefit of these annual outings was time spent learning together whether we were driving, fishing, hiking, building sand castles or relaxing around our campsite every evening. I feel that we passed on our appreciation for and love of the outdoors to our children because they still go camping with friends/family and Hazlon bought our first family cottage in 2002.

Team Schepmyer ROCKS!

Our support for our children is unconditional and infinite. Through years of walking and talking together, our children observed our actions in challenging times and they came to recognize that they can count on our unwavering support. I know this faith in us gave them the confidence to step up and step outside of what was considered the normal paths to take in many areas of life.

This time doing activities together was very important to us because of our weekday schedules. When the girls were very young, Neville and I were rarely at home at the same time. Our schedules revolved around Neville's work hours (3:00 p.m. to 11:00 p.m.) because of the security of his job, its benefits and opportunities for overtime. To accommodate this, I accepted a position with the Toronto District School Board working from 6:00 a.m. to 2:00 p.m. during the week. Fortunately, due to the proximity of our jobs and our schedules, we did not need to pay for childcare. Instead, we arranged to meet in a mall parking lot, where I would take the children from Neville.

One thing we worked hard at maintaining was our Sunday morning family breakfast of bakes and scrambled eggs. In addition to sharing a meal, we almost always played "The Parson's Cat" which is also known as "The Minister's Cat". In the basic version of this word game, all players sit in a circle, and the first player describes the Parson's cat with an adjective beginning with the letter 'A' (for example, "The Parson's cat is an adorable cat"). Each player then does the same, using different adjectives starting with the same letter. Typically, once everyone has done so, the first player describes the cat with an adjective beginning with the letter 'B'. This continues for each letter of the alphabet.

In our house, we kept going around and around the table until someone ran out of novel adjectives starting with letter 'A' and had to move on to adjectives starting with letter 'B'. Our love for that game continued for years especially during breakfast and also during our Sunday afternoon drives. We recognized that Andrew was intellectually gifted when, at just two years old, he joined in the game on a family drive to Ottawa! The love of word games runs deep on Team Schepmyer! *Author's note: My younger brother and I now own our childhood home and my parents live here with me. I can guarantee that part of the book launch celebrations will be a Parson's Cat marathon at Chateau Schepmyer!*

APPENDIX A
How does Haze define her GRIT?

> **From https://growmygrit.com/blog/ (October 2019)**

So I thought it would be helpful for me to describe my own GRIT as an example and as a way for you to get to know more about me! I love to play with words, so I tried to find G, R, I and T words that reflect my default setting when things get tough for me. I want to acknowledge that everyone's version of tough is different; I understand that the challenges people face will vary in complexity and intensity. I'd say that most of the obstacles and challenges I have faced so far are setbacks, detours or full-out roadblocks that I have chosen to navigate.

Using the example of losing what I thought was *the best job ever* this past June, here's how I define my GRIT.

My G is for GRATITUDE because my brain reliably sees how things could be so much worse in the face of bad news, loss or a tough situation. When we got the news about our jobs being cut, my first thoughts were: (i) I'm grateful for three months' notice because some people get walked out or locked out when they lose their jobs; (ii) I'm grateful that I'm the only person in my organization with my job title because I'm not going to be competing with dozens of friends and colleagues for a new job; (iii) I'm grateful that I'm getting a severance package which recognizes my 14 years of service to the organization and I can work right up until September to finish all of my projects on-the-go.

My R is for RESILIENCE because I tend to keep sight of the surface when the flood waters of change start gushing and rushing. My brain is also quick to come up with explanations for tough situations that allow me not to take things personally. When the news came about the cuts, I realized that I'd be losing what I thought was *the best job ever*. However, as I was the only person in my role, I wasn't left wondering why I was losing my job while some of my other colleagues weren't. I believe in abundance and so I figured that there must be another *best job ever* out there for me and I'd just have to find it. Little did I know I'd be the one to create my next *best job ever*! Another thought that crossed my mind was that my brain had been my most important resource on-the-job and it was coming with me, so all would be well in the end.

My I is for IMAGINATION because, whether I like it or not, I imagine scenarios to infinity and beyond. By sifting through those scenarios, I can identify how things might be different and imagine which path will get me closer to where I want to be.

My T is for TIME which I'm very aware is a finite resource. I want to honour all of the feelings that come my way (happy, sad, ecstatic, frustrated, awestruck, disappointed, energized, embarrassed, stoked) but I try to remind myself that any time spent in a negative mindset is cutting into the time I could be spending in a positive place. When things are getting tough for me, I sometimes set myself a time limit. This means I can feel sorry for myself and sulk for two or three more hours and then I'll focus on the next part of my day.

Feel, heal then deal with what's real (i.e., what's happening outside of your mind)! This is my GRIT, what's yours?

About the Author

For as long as she can remember, Hazlon (Haze) Schepmyer has been encouraging people to consider the unique strengths they reliably bring to difficult situations. She became an official Gritty Guru in 2019 after losing the best job ever and then deciding to create the best job ever!

For Haze, the best job EVER is one in which she gets to facilitate conversations that help people to know, grow and show their GRIT (i.e., one's default setting when navigating obstacles and challenges).

Haze has honed her GRIT in various settings over the last three decades and those experiences informed her unique approach to self-exploration and self-discovery. In the last two decades, Haze has given presentations and facilitated workshops across Europe, the United States and Canada.

Haze is currently working on the sequel, *"Too Much GRIT to Quit!"*, which will document and celebrate the incredible stories of many Gritty Gurus from the first year after knowing, growing and showing their GRIT. Share your compass and your story on Instagram or Facebook @growmygrit!

Learn more at growmygrit.com

www.ingramcontent.com/pod-product-compliance
Lightning Source LLC
Chambersburg PA
CBHW020908080526
44589CB00011B/493